GOLF FITNESS

GOLF FITNESS

Play Better,
Play without Pain,
Play Longer,
and Enjoy the Game More

KAREN PALACIOS-JANSEN

and the Editors of *Golf Fitness Magazine*

FOREWORD BY GARY PLAYER

TAYLOR TRADE PUBLISHING
Lanham • New York • Boulder • Toronto • Plymouth, UK

Disclaimer
This book is not intended for the treatment or prevention of disease, nor as a substitute for medical treatment. Any reader should not attempt any programs mentioned herein, without reviewing and consulting with your doctor or health professional. The authors are neither responsible, nor liable for any harm or injury resulting from these programs or the use of the exercises described herein.

Published by Taylor Trade Publishing
An imprint of The Rowman & Littlefield Publishing Group, Inc.
4501 Forbes Boulevard, Suite 200, Lanham, Maryland 20706
http://www.rlpgtrade.com

Estover Road, Plymouth PL6 7PY, United Kingdom

Distributed by National Book Network

British Library Cataloguing in Publication Information Available

Library of Congress Cataloging-in-Publication Data
Palacios-Jansen, Karen.
    Golf fitness : play better, play without pain, play longer and enjoy the game more / Karen Palacios-Jansen and editors of Golf Fitness Magazine.
        p. cm.
    Includes bibliographical references and index.
    ISBN 978-1-58979-611-9 (pbk.) — ISBN 978-1-58979-612-6 (electronic)
    1. Golf—Training. 2. Physical fitness. I. Golf fitness magazine. II. Title.
GV979.T68P35 2011
796.352—dc22   2011012382

♾️™ The paper used in this publication meets the minimum requirements of American National Standard for Information Sciences—Permanence of Paper for Printed Library Materials, ANSI/NISO Z39.48-1992.

Printed in the United States of America

CONTENTS

FOREWORD

I **have always** been an uncompromising proponent of diet, health, and fitness and have long been an advocate of golf being considered not just a pastime, but a sport, and golfers as athletes. Being fit was one of the most important factors in my success. It allowed me to be a better golfer and a more mentally focused player as well. I was not the most naturally gifted player of my generation, but I was the fittest and best prepared—that was my edge. When you prepare your body and mind to become a champion, you will become a champion.

Today fitness has become a part of the game. The shift in attitude toward diet, health, and fitness and away from the belief that golfers did not have to be in good physical shape to win is fantastic for the game and golfers alike. I believe that we are now witnessing a permanent and positive change toward the beliefs that I have had about golf fitness and health for many years, and not just for adult players, but for juniors as well. Even if you are not a competitive golfer, the benefits of proper diet and regular exercise go far beyond your golf game.

I am 75 years old and am still as strong and fit as ever. I exercise every day and am careful with my nutritional intake and still play competitive golf. I regularly break my age in tournament play, a testament to my physical well being. Longevity reflects who I am, and my dedication to health and golf fitness has been the key, not only to my success on the golf course but my success in life.

Becoming a champion golfer presents one of the toughest mental and physical challenges one will ever face. You have to work harder than everyone else and always believe that you will be successful. Diet, health, and fitness are the foundation for success, and if golfers, both professional and amateur, took their health more seriously, they would not only be better players but be able to enjoy the game well into their latter years.

This book presented by *Golf Fitness Magazine* is your opportunity to explore how to implement the benefits of functional golf fitness for a stronger, more agile, and safer body movement for your game. You will immediately see and feel the results toward a positive change in your ability to play. Golf is a sport you can enjoy for a lifetime, and if you keep yourself golf fit, you will be guaranteed lower scores and more enjoyment of your passion for many years to come!

Gary

Gary Player
Golf Fitness Magazine

PREFACE

For centuries, golf was considered a game in which the royal, elite, and privileged participated in a leisurely fashion (or so they thought). Then came advances in golf course design and golf equipment, which increased the demands for physical skill and brought out the likes of Snead, Hogan, Player, Palmer, and Nicklaus. These were probably the first signs that golf had changed from more of a game to a sport, but it wasn't until this past decade that Tiger Woods's influence and domination in professional golf made it clear that fitness, mental focus, nutrition, performance, and golf health are fundamental to playing the sport to the best of one's ability. This influence was the tipping point toward a real and permanent change in the way professionals train today for golf and the way the rest of us will learn, practice, and play for evermore.

As we witness the inspiration of our awesome Tour athletes and combine it with today's advanced research in functional golf fitness, better health, and longevity, we are experiencing an evolutionary transformation in the way the game (or sport as we like to call it) of golf is perceived and understood. Fortunately a paradigm shift has already taken place, and for us enthusiastic golfers, with our large incidence of injury and scoring handicaps that haven't improved for 30 years, we understand now more than ever that conditioning our bodies for golf is the key, the answer, to our woes on the golf course. By improving our athleticism required for golf, we are in turn improving our personal ability, permanently lowering our scores, reducing our risk of golf-related injury, and ultimately finding more joy in our passion.

If you haven't already gotten into improving your level of conditioning for golf, begin by using this book to get a jump start on a better

Golfers are realizing more than ever that total golf game improvement, injury prevention, and lower scores all come from better physical and mental conditioning no matter what your age, handicap, or gender. *Golf Fitness Magazine* is at the forefront of the fitness movement, helping their readers by providing a publication that focuses on total game improvement through physical and mental performance for golfers of all ages.

—STEVE GOMEN, GFM Publisher

game. You will be amazed what dramatic and permanent effects can be realized with a little effort toward golf-specific fitness.

Swing solid and play safe!

Steve Gomen
Publisher
Golf Fitness Magazine

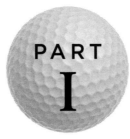

PART

I

THE BODY
AND SWING

CHAPTER 1

INTRODUCTION TO GOLF FITNESS

Twenty years ago, the words *golf and fitness* might have never been used in the same sentence, especially when the majority of golfers were beer-bellied guys riding in carts. Many did not even view golf as a sport, but rather a game played by nonathletes too old or out of shape to play more strenuous sports. This belief changed after Tiger Woods began dominating the world of golf. Through fitness, Tiger Woods completely changed his body and swing. He went from being a thin teenager with a loose, unreliable swing to having the body of an elite athlete with a controlled, powerful swing that has forever changed the game of golf. Legendary golfer Gary Player, with nine major championship wins, credits Woods for revolutionizing the game of golf. Player says that Woods's success has been noticed by the rest of the Tour and is making a big impact on how the game is perceived. "He raised the bar for those on Tour," Player said about Woods.

Ask any Tour player today and most will tell you that they have had to either beef up their fitness routine or start a program all together just to keep from getting lapped by the top players in the world. Padraig Harrington, who won two majors in the 2008 season, the British Open and PGA (Professional Golf Association) Championship, said that Tiger Woods inspired him to work even harder. Many PGA Tour players are also thinking ahead to the Senior PGA Tour, so they are adding fitness to their daily regimens to prevent injury and extend their playing careers. PGA Tour player Retief Goosen, winner of two US Open Championships, credits Woods for inspiring him to get into condition. "I was looking at myself in the mirror and thinking, 'I look a

> If you put the work in, and that means on the range and in the fitness room, it pays off. When you stop working at it, that's when you lose your edge. It's as important what you do on the course as what you do off the course.
>
> **—TIGER WOODS**

bit out of shape,'" Goosen said after winning the Transitions Championship after turning 40 during the year. "I started to work hard in the gym. I feel better about myself and am a lot more consistent. I think the whole Tour has learned a lesson from Tiger." Today, most Tour players have incorporated some sort of fitness program into their lives.

But many golfers will still argue that technology and equipment has changed the game more in the last twenty years than fitness and will point out such players as John Daly and Tim Herron as examples of out-of-shape golfers who still compete. These golfers shrug off the importance of a preround warm-up and opt for a hot dog and beer at the turn for energy while relying on their high-tech drivers and forgiving irons as fixes for their serious swing flaws. These golfers still have the mindset that spending hours on the range beating balls and playing as much as possible with their new equipment, rather than spending some time working on their bodies, will eventually lead to improvement and lower scores. But as the professional ranks have increased their yardage off the tee and improved their control of the ball around the greens exponentially through high-tech equipment and improved fitness, the national handicap, about 19 for the average golfer, has not changed much at all, despite the advancements in equipment. The missing link for these underachieving golfers is fitness. What these golfers don't understand is that even if they were to take lessons with a professional and get out on the course with their new clubs three times a week, if they have not addressed their physical deficiencies, their game may not improve to its full potential and may actually weaken with each hole throughout a round due to fatigue.

Do you have to be super flexible like Camilo Villegas, bench press 200 pounds like Tiger Woods, or do triathlons like Lorena Ochoa to be in golf shape? Not necessarily. Golf fitness is not about bodybuilding or even losing weight, it is about playing better golf. Being in "golf shape" means being able to play 18 holes without getting tired or losing concentration, being flexible enough to make a complete shoulder turn, or just being able to swing a club without pain.

Golf, although not thought of as a strenuous activity, requires a higher level of fitness than most people would think. In a single round, a golfer will take an average of 300 swings (including practice swings) and walk 7,000 to 8,000 yards, the equivalent of four to five miles. Swinging a club over and over again twists the neck, back, shoulders, and arms unnaturally, and the physical stress loads become substantial. "In the last decade, golfers have come to grips with the fact that strength, flexibility, and overall fitness play a critical role in the game. Stronger, fitter, more flexible athletes hit a ball farther and straighter, have better touch around the greens, and respond better under pressure in the closing holes than do their weaker counterparts. Golf is more than a game; it is a sport and, as is the case in all athletic sports, fitness is crucial. So being fit for the game of golf is the future," says PGA teaching professional and *Golf Fitness Magazine* contributor Cindy Reid.

Do you need to start pumping iron or jogging to get into golf shape? Although those things will help, they are not necessary to improve your game. There are many other simple things you can do that don't even involve breaking a sweat to improve your golf game. If you already work out, you can add a few golf-specific exercises to your routine that can make huge improvements to your game. If you have never worked out, you can start by working new habits into your daily life, like warming up before a round or spending a few minutes a day stretching. Paying attention to your diet can also help you play better golf. Managing your food intake and adding certain nutrients to your diet can help you concentrate and focus more on the golf course.

Golf fitness is about making small changes in your life and daily routine to improve your golf game dramatically. Golf fitness is for players of all ages and levels. You can make dramatic changes to your game no matter what shape your body is in or what level of player you are. Whether you are a low-handicap player who plays in high-level competitions or a weekend golfer with a wicked slice, golf fitness can always help improve your level of play. Junior golfers can also benefit from incorporating golf fitness into their daily routines by building a foundation of good habits, like stretching and warming up before play, that will last a lifetime.

This book is packed with many of the essentials you will need to continue to improve your game throughout your lifetime, including advice from leading golf fitness professionals to help you improve your strength, flexibility, and endurance; tips to help you prevent injury; pointers to help you concentrate and focus better on the golf course; and suggestions to help you improve your score. This is a different way to learn the game of golf. We believe fundamentals and swing mechanics are interconnected and important to your game as well, but this book focuses on improving your body and mind to play better golf.

Many of you may be eager yet unsure of how to start a golf fitness program. We at GFM have assembled the most important advice and techniques to guide you in the process of starting a program to help you play your best golf. Beginning with how to assess your body

10 REASONS TO START
A GOLF FITNESS PROGRAM

1. *Golf fitness helps you hit it longer.* Doing golf-specific strength and speed exercises is one of the fastest ways to improve your distance off the tee.

2. *Golf fitness helps you hit more solid golf shots.* When you improve your fitness, you improve your body's ability to move fluidly and effectively, therefore delivering more power to the ball with less effort. Improving your mobility, strength, and balance helps you execute your golf swing more efficiently to make better and more consistent contact with the ball.

3. *Golf fitness helps protect you from injury.* Last year golfers suffered approximately 35,000 injuries that required a trip to the emergency room or doctor, according to the National Safety Council. Strengthening your muscles, especially in your body's midsection or core, offers protection to the rest of your body. A strong core improves the performance of your other muscles, therefore helping to prevent chronic nagging and acute injuries.

4. *Golf fitness helps you play longer.* Being fit is the key to golf longevity. As we age, we lose flexibility and strength, so the more fit you are, the more you can ward off the negative effects of aging.

5. *Golf fitness helps you perform at your peak.* When your body and mind are fit and strong, you are able to perform at your highest level.

6. *Golf fitness helps save your joints.* Arthritis affects 50 percent of Americans over the age of 65. It is most common in the hips, spine, and knees. Maintaining strength in your muscles and joints helps you swing better and prevent potential injuries.

7. *Golf fitness helps you concentrate and focus better.* Being physically fit helps you be more alert and ward off fatigue so you can concentrate and focus better and longer while you play. One area recreational golfers most often neglect is their nutritional intake before and especially during a round of golf. Managing your food intake and adding certain nutrients to your diet not only help you concentrate and focus more on the golf course but also keep your heartbeat steady as you make an important shot or putt, help your muscles fire faster for more power, help you fight fatigue so you can play and practice longer, and even keep your blood pressure down so you can keep your cool after a bad shot.

8. *Golf fitness helps protect your back.* The golf swing is one of the most stressful movements on the lower back. Becoming more physically fit helps protect your back and prevents potential injuries. By eliminating those nagging aches and pains before,

during, or after a round of golf, you can practice and play more often.

9. *Golf fitness helps combat chronic diseases.* Worried about heart disease? Hoping to prevent osteoporosis? Regular exercise helps prevent or manage these diseases and maintains your blood pressure and cholesterol levels.

10. *Golf fitness helps you sleep better.* Struggling to fall asleep or stay asleep? Becoming physically active helps you sleep better, and a good night's sleep improves your concentration and focus on the golf course.

to identify your strengths and weaknesses so that you can choose the best exercises specific to your needs, we then show how these physical limitations may be affecting your golf swing and what you can do about it. We demonstrate how to warm up before you play to shave strokes off your score and prevent injury. We also provide exercises that will help improve your range of motion to get you into those positions your golf professional has been trying to get you in all these years. Want to know how Tour professionals work out? We show you the fitness routines of some of the world's best players. We illustrate how making the right choices in terms of preround meals and on-course snacks can help you concentrate and focus better. We give tips and techniques so you can take your game to the next level by working on your mental game. Committing to golf fitness will allow you to achieve your personal best game. Let's get started.

CHAPTER 2

SWING FAULTS

Are you frustrated because you take lessons to improve your swing and practice regularly without positive results? Do you try to make a bigger shoulder turn, but no matter how hard you try, you just can't get into the position your pro shows you? Have you been told that you have swing faults, but you just can't seem to correct them on your own? Your swing faults may be from physical limitations. Your body, because of lack of flexibility, mobility, and/or strength, is holding you back from correcting your swing faults and playing your best golf. Most golf professionals will tell you that such common swing faults as poor posture and lack of rotation are from physical limitations, and until you address those limitations you may never improve.

The purpose of this chapter is to help you understand and identify swing faults and the physical limitations that may cause them. Swing faults, which are technical flaws in your golf swing, can be caused by physical limitations or such improper swing mechanics as lack of strength and inflexibility in crucial areas of the body. Flexibility, strength, coordination, balance, and stability in your golf-specific muscles are imperative in making a good golf swing and playing your best.

Physical limitations or weaknesses can affect the way you swing a golf club. For example, if you have tight hamstring muscles, it will be difficult for you to maintain the correct amount of spine angle during the swing. You may "come out of the shot" or "stand up" through impact, which can cause topped or weak shots. If you lack strength or flexibility in your hips or buttocks, you may not be able to shift your weight properly and as a result lose power and consistency.

Identifying your swing faults and physical limitations is absolutely necessary in building a fundamentally sound golf swing. Identifying and correcting your swing faults and physical limitations should be a focal point in your golf-specific fitness program. Playing golf with physical limitations or common swing flaws can cause serious injury to the most vulnerable parts of your body, including the lower back, neck, elbows, and wrists. Identifying and correcting swing flaws will not only improve your golf game, but also help you prevent the most common golf injuries.

Our GFM team has assembled a list of the eight most common swing faults. These include the following:

1. poor posture
2. reverse pivot
3. sway
4. loss of spine angle
5. lack of rotation
6. coming over the top
7. early release
8. lack of weight shift

Identifying your swing faults will help you and your golf teacher or golf fitness professional design a golf fitness program to fit your specific needs.

SWING FAULT #1: POOR POSTURE

If you setup correctly, there's a good chance you'll hit a reasonable shot, even if you make a mediocre swing. If you set up to the ball poorly, you'll hit a lousy shot, even if you make the greatest swing in the world.

—JACK NICKLAUS

The following six physical limitations can contribute to poor posture:

1. tight chest muscles
2. limited range of motion in the upper back
3. weak neck muscles
4. tight hips
5. weak gluteal muscles (buttocks) and abdominal muscles
6. lack of pelvic tilt

The cornerstone of a good golf swing is the establishment of the ideal posture at address position. Ideally, a golfer should strive to attain a neutral alignment of the spine, where the neck, middle back, and lower back align properly without excessive arching or curvature. A poor setup forces you to make compensations in your swing, so it is important to find the correct setup for your swing and learn to repeat it. Most high-handicappers and even some low-handicappers and professionals make common mistakes in their setups that cause them to hit bad shots, develop bad habits, and wreak havoc on their bodies. Let's take a look at some of the most common problems and why they occur.

S-Posture

S-posture is the anatomical term referring to an increased curve in the thoracic spine (middle to upper back) and lumbar spine (lower back) (see figure 2.1). The spine maintains a normal curvature, and this natural bend works as a shock absorber, distributing the stress that occurs during daily movement. S-posture is characterized by excessive curvatures in the spine at address position. As the golfer sets up to the ball, his or her spine may have too much curvature, creating the appearance of the letter "S." S-posture can disrupt the golf swing sequence due to muscle imbalances, resulting in unwanted compensatory movements of the golf swing. It also hinders proper rotation and mobility of the spine's joints due to less than optimal joint position. When this occurs, golfers tend to lift their torso up, losing spine angle to subconsciously try to complete their backswing. They will also try to overswing with their arms and tend to come over the top.

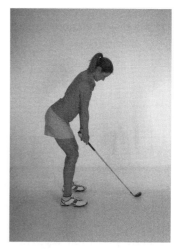

FIGURE 2.1

C-Posture

C-posture is the anatomical term referring to an increased middle/upper back curve (thoracic kyphosis) (see figure 2.2). Kyphosis is characterized by excessive outward curvature of the spine, causing hunching of the back. In golf terms, C-posture is used to describe a posture that occurs when the shoulders are slumped forward at address position and there is a definitive roundness in the back from the tailbone upward to the back of the neck. It is common in individuals who have classic, poor, or slumped posture.

If a golfer has this type of posture, it will limit the extent to which the torso and shoulders are able to rotate on the backswing. The upper back is designed to rotate and is the primary area of the spine that rotates the shoulders, while the lower back rotates minimally. The lower back is designed to flex and extend. The thoracic spine (upper back) can optimally rotate only when hunching over is eliminated. To experience this, sit down and hunch over and try to rotate your shoulders. Then

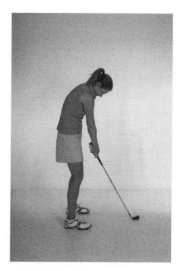

FIGURE 2.2

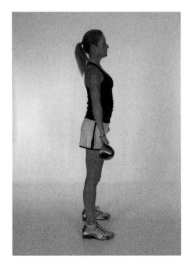

POSTURE EXERCISE

Most people do not have good posture and are unaware of postural issues that may affect their golf swing. Do you know what your posture looks like? With a friend watching, walk in place, then stop after three steps. Have your friend stand at your side and look at your posture. Ask them to compare it to the pictures of good posture, S-posture, and C-posture. Your golf shot can be greatly affected by your S-posture or C-posture. Figure 2.3 is an example of good posture. Top assume the proper posture, imagine a straight line passing from your ankles through your shoulders and ears.

FIGURE 2.3

try to rotate when you sit up straight and the spine is aligned properly. The shoulder/torso rotation increases dramatically.

This physical limitation will cause a golfer to be hunched over the ball at address position. As a result, the player will find it difficult to maintain posture as he or she swings the club back, usually resulting in a short, tight backswing. The arms may bend to get the club to parallel. The golfer with C-posture may also raise the entire body when starting the swing to gain momentum to swing the club to the top of the swing. This posture can simply be the result of a poor set-up position and can be easily corrected by physically adjusting the posture to a more neutral spine.

Unfortunately, the majority of C-postures are caused by a series of muscle imbalances and joint restrictions developed from years of poor posture or lack of exercise. Many of our daily activities, for example, sitting at a desk typing at a computer, driving in the car, or sitting on the couch watching television, contribute to poor posture and muscle imbalances. Research shows that a C-posture is a result of muscle and joint imbalance. If the imbalances are slight, they can be corrected by performing strength and flexibility exercises.

SWING FAULT #2: REVERSE PIVOT

Physical limitations that can cause a reverse pivot include the following:

1. inability to separate the upper body from the lower body
2. limited spinal mobility
3. limited trunk rotation
4. limited internal hip rotation
5. lack of core stability
6. S-posture
7. lack of lower body strength
8. lack of balance

The reverse pivot occurs in the backswing when the golfer straightens his or her back leg and shifts their body weight to the front leg and the upper body tilts toward the target instead of away from the target (see figure 2.4 for an example of what a reverse pivot looks like). This motion inhibits the amount of torque a golfer can create on the backswing because they cannot rotate their body, forcing them to make compensations in their swing on the downswing. This reverse pivot, or reverse weight shift, as it is sometimes called, is due to compensation caused by weakness of the back leg's hip and thigh muscles, specifically the gluteus maximus muscles (buttocks) and quadriceps.

If these muscles are weak, the golfer will not be able to physically handle shifting their weight correctly onto their back leg on the backswing. The golfer will tend to straighten the back leg by locking the knee, which helps support the body weight, and then the golfer will tend to shift the weight to the front leg to maintain balance. A reverse pivot forces the golfer to start the downswing with the upper body, denying them the leverage to maximize clubhead speed. A reverse pivot will also put a tremendous amount of pressure on the lower spine, which can cause pain or injury.

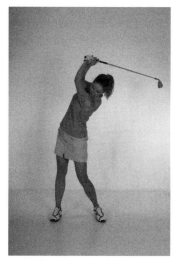

FIGURE 2.4

SWING FAULT # 3: SWAY

The following four physical limitations can cause sway:

1. weak gluteal muscles (buttocks)
2. tight hips
3. lack of spinal mobility
4. lack of trunk mobility

Sway is a golf term that indicates a sideways movement of the lower body on the backswing (see figure 2.5 for a demonstration of what sway

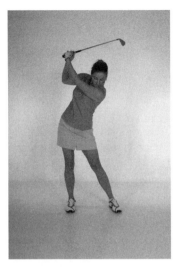

FIGURE 2.5

looks like). Ideally, the hips are to turn during the backswing, with only a slight lateral motion. A sway indicates excessive lateral motion with the lower body. A sway also limits the weight shift and may cause the golfer to move his or her head off the ball. Golfers that sway may also lock or straighten their back knee as they start the backswing. This motion inhibits the amount of torque a golfer can create on the backswing because they cannot rotate their body, forcing them to make compensations in their swing on the downswing.

A sway, whether it is on the backswing or downswing (a downswing sway is sometimes called "slide") can be directly attributed to weakness or inhibition of the gluteal muscles (buttocks) or hips. The buttocks are the principal muscles used in supporting the body on one leg. If they are weak or there is a delay in contraction of these muscles, the pelvis will sway in the direction of the loading of the weight, and there is a tremendous amount of stored energy lost. If these muscles are weak, the golfer will slide to shift their weight on the backswing and downswing instead of rotating the lower body.

One of the most widely used terms in golf instruction is the idea of the "one-piece" takeaway. Many golf instructors believe that the club, arms, and body move away from the ball in a solid one-piece motion. But if you have some sort of physical limitation in your hips, knees, or torso, practicing this concept can cause you to sway.

SWING FAULT #4: LOSS OF SPINE ANGLE

Physical limitations that can cause loss of spine angle include the following:

1. limited core stability
2. weak gluteal muscles (buttocks)
3. lack of spinal mobility
4. tight hamstrings
5. tight chest muscles
6. tight and weak back muscles

Ideally, the amount of spine angle you create at your address position should remain constant throughout your golf swing. If the angle is compromised at any point in the swing, for example, if you raise up as you swing the club back or you straighten your body as you strike the ball, you will not be able to maintain the club on the proper swing plane (see figure 2.6 for a demonstration of what loss of spine angle looks like).

Maintaining a constant spine angle in the golf swing is essential to solid, consistent ball contact. Any upward or downward movement with the body causes a chain reaction of compensations that adversely affect the mechanics of the golf swing, including inconsistent ball contact and loss of balance and power, and greatly increases your chance of injury. If a golfer's abdominal muscles are inhibited or weak or the thoracic spine (upper back) does not have proper flexibility, he or she will be unable to maintain the correct spine angle throughout the swing due to subconscious compensation by lifting up to complete the golf swing.

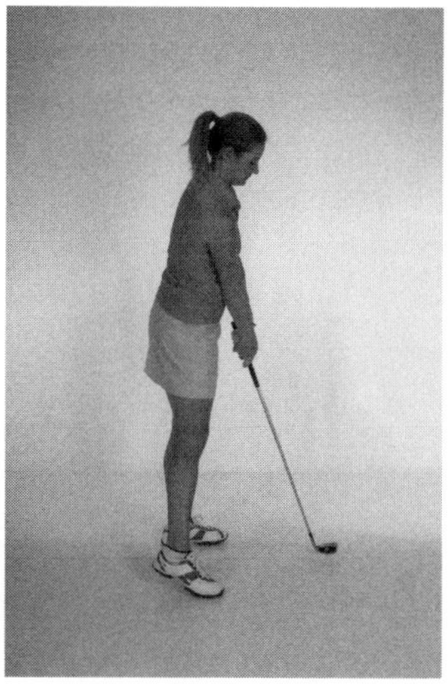

FIGURE 2.6

THE OVERHEAD DEEP SQUAT

Statistical research at the Titleist Performance Institute has found several correlations between the overhead deep squat and the golf swing. If a golfer is unable to perform a full deep squat with their heels on the ground, it can be difficult for them to maintain their posture during the downswing. Loss of spine angle, where the action of thrusting the lower body toward the golf ball and straightening the torso during the downswing, sometimes called "early extension," is common.

SWING FAULT #5: LACK OF ROTATION

The following eight physical limitations can cause lack of rotation:

1. inability to separate the upper body from the lower body
2. weak gluteus medius muscles (buttocks)
3. limited hip rotation
4. weak abdominal muscles
5. tight upper back muscles
6. lack of shoulder rotation
7. lack of trunk rotation
8. lack of spine mobility

Most golf instructors agree that to achieve maximum power, you need to rotate your shoulders to a 90-degree angle and your hips to a 45-degree angle in relation to the golf ball at address position. Most

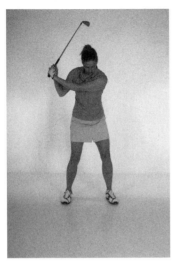

FIGURE 2.7

golfers never achieve a complete shoulder, torso, and hip turn, resulting in a reduced or shortened backswing (see figure 2.7 for an example of lack of shoulder rotation). Lack of rotation may lead to a variety of compensations, including lifting or bending the arms to complete the backswing, swaying, and overuse of the hands and wrists at impact.

Lack of shoulder, torso, and hip rotation can be caused by weaknesses in the internal and external oblique muscles and lack of flexibility of the thoracic spine. The ability to separate your upper body from your lower body allows your shoulders to rotate around your spine without altering your original posture. If you can't turn your upper body separately from your lower body, you will have limited trunk rotation. Lack of rotation or limited rotation can also be caused by underuse of internal/external oblique and hip muscles. Because most of us lead a professional lifestyle, sitting behind a desk for hours at a time or sitting behind the wheel of a car in traffic, most people do not rotate their upper bodies during the day. These muscles tend to go to sleep or become inhibited.

Another reason for limited rotation can be lack of flexibility and mobility of the upper back. If there is too much curve in the upper back and overall poor posture of the spine, where the neck, middle back, and lower back are not aligned, torso rotation will be limited.

SWING FAULT #6: COMING OVER THE TOP

Physical limitations that can cause coming over the top include the following:

1. tight neck muscles
2. C-posture
3. tight hips
4. limited hip rotation
5. weak core stability
6. weak gluteal muscles (buttocks)
7. weak abdominal muscles
8. inability to separate the upper body from the lower body

The phrase "coming over the top" is used to describe the movement of the club as it travels through the downswing. It occurs because of an overdominance of the upper body as the downswing is initiated. As a result, the club is thrown outside of the intended swing plane, with the clubhead approaching the ball from an outside path (figure 2.8

illustrates what it looks like when a golfer comes over the top). This creates a pull if the clubface is square or a slice if the clubface is open. This fault will cause loss of power and limit the ability to control the ball flight. In addition, this motion can impart a left-to-right spin (for right-handed golfers) on the ball flight, causing a slice.

Ideally, you want to initiate the downswing with the lower body so that the club and arms can drop into the correct position, allowing the clubhead to approach the ball from an inside path. The correct sequence of motion on the downswing is determined by the golfer's ability to disassociate the lower body from the upper body so that the lower body can lead on the downswing. A golfer who tends to come over the top usually has limited trunk to pelvis separation caused by reduced spinal and hip mobility. The result is that the upper body dominates the initiation of the downswing.

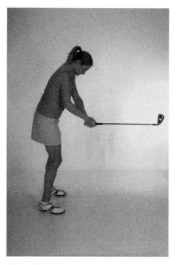

FIGURE 2.8

Limited weight shift toward the lead leg can also reduce the lower body's contribution to power generation in the swing, thereby forcing the golfer to produce excessive power in their upper body or by throwing the club over the top. Also, if the neck muscles are tight and the shoulders are raised, forward, and tense, an over-the-top move on the downswing is inevitable.

SWING FAULT #7: EARLY RELEASE

The following five physical limitations can cause early release:

1. lack of hip mobility
2. lack of ankle mobility
3. lack of core stabilization
4. lack of hand and wrist strength and mobility
5. tight hips

All good players have one position in the golf swing that's similar despite their very different swings. This position is impact. Good players retain their wrist cock through the hitting area so that their lead wrist is bowed and their back wrist is extended and both hands are slightly in front of the golf ball at the strike. This is often called a "late hit" or "clubhead lag," and good players use both to create a tremendous amount of clubhead speed and power in their swings.

High-handicappers tend to do the opposite at impact. Instead of a late hit, they actually execute what's called an "early release." They scoop

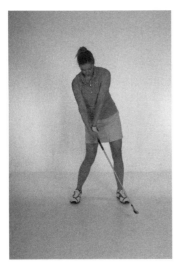

FIGURE 2.9

the ball at impact because they lose the lag too early in the downswing. Instead of having a flat lead wrist and their hands ahead of the ball at impact, they have a collapsed lead wrist with their hands behind the ball at impact (see figure 2.9 for a demonstration of an early release). As such, they suffer a tremendous loss of power and direction and end up with a very weak hit. Golfers with this problem tend to hit the ball better with their woods than their irons, because the ball is teed up and they can get away with scooping or hitting up on the ball. To hit solid irons shots and better drives more consistently, however, it's necessary to hit down with a flat lead wrist that's ahead of the ball at impact.

To create a late hit and eliminate the early release, you must sequence the swing so that your hands, your wrists, and the clubhead arrive at impact in the correct order. There are many causes of an early release, including limitations in the wrists or wrist injury; faulty sequencing of the swing due to such swing faults as reverse pivot, sway, and coming over the top; and lack of strength in the upper and lower body.

Good wrist flexibility is essential for setting the club to create angle in the wrists and maintaining that angle during the downswing. The back wrist must have good extension, the left wrist must be able to flex, and both wrists must have ample radial deviation to be able to hinge the club. Second, strong forearm and grip strength are important to set and hold the club properly. Third, as with most upper body swing faults, any dysfunction in the lower body can be the root cause. In other words, if the lower body is not initiating the sequence of power, the upper body will try to compensate to make up for the missing lower body. Many times a golfer with an early release will have very little body rotation and weight shift on the downswing, and as a result, the large centripetal force of the club will cause the hands to stop at the moment of impact, while the clubhead continues moving, resulting in a scoop motion.

SWING FAULT #8: LACK OF WEIGHT SHIFT

Physical limitations that can cause lack of weight shift include the following:

1. lack of strength in gluteus medius and gluteus maximus muscles (buttocks)
2. lack of balance
3. inability to separate the upper body from the lower body
4. limited hip rotation

To get power and distance and strike the ball solidly, you must create a powerful backswing coil by getting your weight onto your back leg at the top of your swing and then shifting your weight entirely onto the front leg on the downswing. Coiling results from turning the upper body against the resistance of the lower body and then unleashing the energy stored in the coil by shifting all your weight on the downswing. Look at any good golfer and you will see that they finish with all their weight shifted onto their front leg.

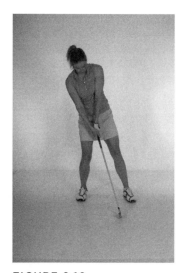

FIGURE 2.10

The initial phase of the downswing begins with the shifting of the lower body, followed by the rotation of the upper body. A typical high-handicap player tends to do the opposite. He or she will rotate their upper body to start the downswing and, as a result, not be able to shift their weight completely on the downswing, finishing the swing with most of his or her weight on the back leg instead of the front leg (figure 2.10 illustrates a lack of weight shift). These errors result in the clubhead approaching the ball on an outside path, causing lack of power and inconsistent ball contact. The inability to optimally fire muscles and utilize the hips and legs in the golf swing are the main causes of lack of weight shift. The lack of power production from the lower body forces the upper body to work harder and overcompensate.

The inability to separate the pelvis from the torso will also cause early initiation of the upper body in the golf swing. This will produce a golf swing dominated by the upper body. If a golfer is not strong enough to handle the weight transfer from the back leg to the front leg, he or she will overcompensate and end up with all their weight on the back leg, causing inconsistent ball contact and a loss of distance.

SUMMARY

Most of these eight common swing faults, if not all, are caused by physical limitations, and many of them are the leading causes of most golf-related injuries. Corrective exercises can eliminate physical limitations and help strengthen golf-specific muscles. Fortunately, correcting these swing faults involves doing common exercises, so when you perform exercises to correct your posture, you will also be correcting other swing faults, including coming over the top and loss of spine angle. In the next chapter, we will perform a basic golf fitness screen to evaluate your physical fitness and determine your physical limitations, strengths, and weaknesses. As you continue to read, you will find many golf-specific exercises designed by our GFM team to help you improve your physical limitations and develop your body for a better golf swing.

CHAPTER 3

ASSESSING YOUR GOLF ABILITY

According to golf fitness professional and GFM contributor Rob Mottram, 75 percent of golfers lack the physical ability to perform the proper body movement to carry out a mechanically correct golf swing. In the late 1980s, Mottram helped develop the Centinela Hospital Fitness Institute's Golf Performance Evaluation, which is given to professional and amateur golfers to assess their level of fitness and wellness as it relates to the game of golf. This evaluation is still in use today. Mottram's team determined that indentifying areas of weakness or lack of mobility is helpful in implementing the proper exercises to improve golf ability and reduce the risk of injury.

Why are these evaluations so important? If it can be determined that you have a certain physical limitation, a golf instructor can work with your swing to help you learn the necessary movements to correct your swing fault. Until you are able to make your body move into certain positions, you will never achieve the swing he or she is attempting to teach you. Worse yet, with the forces generated during the golf swing, improper body movements can result in serious injury. But there is good news. It's not a matter of looking like Tiger Woods to achieve a proper body movement. It is a matter of simply understanding where you might need the increased flexibility or strength. Then it is a matter of putting in a little extra time working on the right things. Your chances of playing better, playing longer, and avoiding injury are greatly improved.

Golf is a highly skilled activity requiring high speed and high range of motion. Most golfers are not physically capable of performing the

Far too often we blame a poor shot on our equipment or not being able to perform a move learned from a golf pro, when actually the culprit is often our physical limitations that prevent us from making a good swing and shot.

—GFM

required movements involved in a mechanically correct golf swing. These limitations often lead to unnecessary stress on various joints and muscles, especially in the lower back, which can cause common golf-related injuries.

To best determine how to reach your fitness goals, you first need to figure out where you are physically. A fitness evaluation is the first step in building a golf fitness program. Identifying and correcting your physical limitations should be a focal point in your golf-specific fitness program.

Even PGA Tour professionals go through evaluations to determine their strengths and weaknesses. PGA Tour professional Trevor Immelman, working with his trainer and GFM contributor Dave Herman, discovered through a golf-specific fitness evaluation that his strongest assets create one of his greatest weaknesses from a technical standpoint. "I have very strong hips, glutes, and legs," says the 2008 Masters champion. "That's why I can create a lot of speed and hit the ball so far, particularly for such a small guy." Herman says that this technically hinders him, because his hips move very fast. Consequently, Immelman concentrates on his rhythm while on the golf course to balance his strength training in the gym, says Herman.

A basic golf-specific screen gives you key information about your physical condition. For you and your fitness professional to design a golf-specific exercise program, it is important to have a plan. With a golf-specific fitness screen, you will be able to determine any physical limitations that may be affecting your performance on the golf course. Identifying your specific strengths and weaknesses will help you in determining what specific exercises you should be performing. "Every once in a while there is a discovery or technological breakthrough in the game of golf that truly makes the game more enjoyable for everyone. Some examples are the modern golf ball and the new hybrid golf clubs that make hitting out of the rough as easy as cutting through a stick of butter. These are all wonderful advances in equipment and golf technology. But in reality, are these breakthroughs really making us better golfers, or are they just making it easier for us to hit golf shots with the same old golf swing—a swing less efficient than what we are actually capable of executing? But physical screens can help improve our bodies to help us swing better," says Steve Gomen, GFM publisher.

The basic golf-specific screen examines the areas involved with the golf swing, including balance; flexibility and strength in the lower body; rotational capacity and strength in the torso and shoulders; and strength and flexibility in the upper body, including the forearms and wrists.[1]

THE BASIC GOLF-SPECIFIC FITNESS SCREEN

1. The Overhead Deep Squat to Test Lower Body Strength and Stability

This test measures the overall mobility in your legs, ankles, shoulders, and spine. If you are unable to perform this test, it is likely that you will not be able to maintain your spine angle throughout your downswing. The natural tendency is to thrust your hips toward the ball at the start of the downswing, thus pulling yourself up and out of the shot and causing an array of errant shots and loss of power. Low results in the overhead deep squat test may be related to C- and S-postures and lack of rotation.

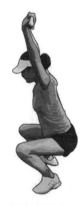

FIGURE 3.1

HOW TO PERFORM THE TEST

- Standing in your golf address position, place a club behind your back or simply raise your arms above your head while holding a golf club.
- Perform a squat as you attempt to maintain your original spine angle.
- Keep your arms raised over your head, knees aligned over your feet, and heels planted on the ground.
- Maintain your balance. See figure 3.1.

Scoring Your Results

1 point
If the club you are holding up above your head falls forward at any time. If your heels raise up off the ground, your feet rotate out as you squat, you cannot bend your hips past your knees, you lose your spine angle, or you lose your balance.

2 points
If you can maintain the club above your head as you squat down and stand back up again. If your heels stay on the ground, but your knees do not stay over your feet or you cannot squat down so that your hips are lower than your knees.

3 points
If you can maintain the club above your head as you squat down and stand back up again. If you can keep your heels

down while you squat down so that your hips are lower than your knees and you are able to keep your knees aligned over your feet.

If you scored less than 2 points, consider improving your upper and lower body strength and stability.

2. The Straight Leg Raise to Test Lower Body Flexibility

This test measures the mobility in your hamstrings and lower back, but it can also detect certain problems or stiffness in your hips that can limit a proper set-up for your full swing or putting stroke. If you are unable to perform this test, you will not be able to maintain your posture (body angles) throughout your swing, which will make it difficult to keep the club on plane. Low test results may also be related to loss of power, loss of posture, and swaying.

HOW TO PERFORM THE TEST

- Lie on your back with both legs and your head flat on the ground. Have a partner place a driver shaft perpendicular to the ground on the outside of your right leg, halfway between your hip and knee.
- Pull your toes toward you and proceed to lift your leg, keeping your knee straight. Your head, hips, and left leg should remain flat on the floor. A golf ball can be placed under your left knee to prevent you from moving your hips or back (see figure 3.2). Complete this movement three times.
- Repeat the test with your left leg.

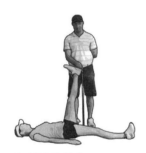

FIGURE 3.2

Scoring Your Results

1 point	If you can only lift your leg at a 45-degree angle.
2 points	If you can lift your leg up parallel to the shaft.
3 points	If you can lift your leg up past the shaft.

If you scored less than 2 points, consider working on your lower body flexibility.

3. The Half-Kneeling Rotation Test

This test measures the overall flexibility between your upper and lower body, along with your core stability. Having good separation between your upper and lower body facilitates greater speed and power in your golf swing. Limited separation can result in a number of swing faults, including too much lateral movement (sway or slide) and loss of posture.

HOW TO PERFORM THE TEST

- Crisscross two golf clubs so that they form four 45-degree angles and look like the letter "X."
- Squat over the crisscrossed golf clubs on your right knee, with your left foot and knee creating a straight line, one in front of the other.
- Place another golf club in the center of your back, locked in with your elbows.
- From this position, keeping your head facing forward, attempt to rotate your shoulders to the left so that the club behind your back matches the club on the ground. See figure 3.3.
- Repeat this exercise on the opposite side.

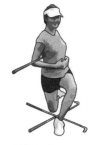

FIGURE 3.3

Scoring Your Results

1 point   If you lose your balance or cannot rotate your upper body.

2 points   If you can rotate your body but the club behind your back does not match the club on the ground.

3 points   If you can rotate your upper body so that the club behind your back matches the club that lies on the ground.

If you scored less than 2 points, consider working on increasing the overall flexibility of your upper body and lower body.

4. The Pelvic Tilt Test

This test measures the range of motion in your lower back and reveals your capacity to engage your abdominal and gluteal muscles. To transfer power from your lower body to your upper body in the golf swing, the ability to control your pelvis is imperative in adding power to your swing and limiting the chances of injury to your lower back. Low test results may also be related to S-posture, loss of posture, and lack of rotation.

HOW TO PERFORM THE TEST

- Get yourself into your golf posture, arms across your chest and your back in a neutral or flat position.

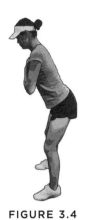

FIGURE 3.4

- Once you have established a neutral starting position, begin tilting your pelvis backwards, arching your lower back as far back as possible without moving your head.
- Upon completion of this movement, tilt your pelvis forward as far as possible, removing the arch in your lower back (see figure 3.4).
- The forward and backward movement of your pelvis should be smooth and continuous, without any shaking motion.

Scoring Your Results

1 point	If you cannot tilt your pelvis forward or arch your back.
2 points	If you feel any shaking motion while you move your pelvis back and forth.
3 points	If you can smoothly tilt your pelvis forward and arch your back without difficulty.

If you scored less than 2 points, you are not using certain abdominal and gluteal muscles on a daily basis that are vital in performing a golf swing.

5. The Single-Leg Balance Test

This test measures your ability to stay balanced throughout your golf swing. If you are unable to perform this test, it is likely that you will have difficulty holding a balanced finish and will be limited in the amount of force you can apply to the golf ball while maintaining good fundamentals.

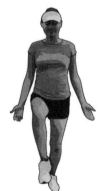

FIGURE 3.5

HOW TO PERFORM THE TEST

- Stand facing forward with your arms extended out by your sides.
- Raise your right knee off of the ground so that your foot is six to eight inches off the ground.
- Hold this position for as long as you can (see figure 3.5).
- Repeat this exercise on the opposite leg.
- Repeat this same exercise with your eyes closed.

Scoring Your Results

1 point	If you can stand on one leg with your eyes open for at least 30 seconds.
2 points	If you can stand on one leg with your eyes closed for at least 15 seconds.

3 points   If you can stand on one leg with your eyes closed for more
            that 30 seconds.

If you scored less than 2 points, consider improving your balance.

6. The Wrist Flexibility and Strength Test

This test measures the strength and flexibility in your wrists. If you are unable to perform this test, it is likely that you will have difficulty hinging the club properly on the backswing and maintaining a flat lead wrist on the moment of impact, resulting in an early release of the club or a scooping motion with the hands and wrists limiting the amount of force you can apply to the ball at impact. Weak wrists are also associated with numerous injuries, including tendonitis.

HOW TO PERFORM THE TEST

- Stand up straight with your arms hanging straight down at your sides.
- Hold a club in your right hand at the end of the grip.
- Slowly move the club up and down by flexing and extending your wrists.
- If you can perform 10 repetitions with one club, add as many clubs as you can until you cannot lift the clubs.
- Repeat the exercise with the other wrist.

Scoring Your Results

1 point   If you can only raise one club up and down for 10 repetitions or less.
2 points   If you can raise two clubs up and down for one repetition or more.
3 points   If you can raise three or more clubs up and down for more than one repetition.

If you scored less than 2 points, consider increasing the strength and flexibility in your wrists.

Scoring

Overhead Deep Squat to Test Lower Body Strength and Stability Score	_____
Straight Leg Raise to Test Lower Body Flexibility Score	_____
Half-Kneeling Rotation Test Score	_____
Pelvic Tilt Test Score	_____
Single-Leg Balance Test Score	_____
Wrist Flexibility and Strength Test Score	_____
Total Score	_____/18

Evaluating Your Results

16–18 POINTS: OPTIMAL GOLF SPECIFIC FITNESS RATING

Congratulations, you passed the basic golf-specific fitness screen. Continue to maintain your fitness level. Remember that flexibility and strength decline with age, so work to maintain this level of fitness by doing the exercises and drills from this book. There should be no physical reason that your swing and game cannot improve. Assess your swing mechanics, scoring statistics, and mental attitude to determine which areas of your game to work on to improve your score. If you scored less than 2 points in any one area of the test, pay special attention to that area of the body.

12–15 POINTS: AVERAGE GOLF SPECIFIC FITNESS RATING

Your fitness level may need some improvement. Striving to improve your fitness level will not only help improve your golf game, but greater fitness will help you prevent injuries and extend your golf career. There may be a physical limitation that is holding you back from playing your best golf. Consider improving your fitness level through a proper training program like the one advised in this book. If you scored less than 2 points in any one area of the test, pay special attention to that area of the body.

12 POINTS OR LESS: BELOW-AVERAGE FITNESS RATING

Do not be discouraged. Although you may not be as fit as you could be, you could see a considerable amount of improvement in your golf game just by adding a few golf-specific exercises. You can overcome your physical limitations by beginning a fitness program to improve your strength and flexibility like the one advised in this book. If you scored less than 2 points in any one area of the test, pay special attention to those areas of the body.

THE ADVANCED GOLF-SPECIFIC POWER SCREEN

Elite athletes have been incorporating "plyometric" or explosive power exercises into their fitness routines for years. Plyometrics is a type of exercise training designed to produce fast, powerful movements and improve the function of the nervous system, generally for the purpose of improving performance in sports.

Professional golfers are now incorporating such explosive power exercises as plyometrics specific to the golf swing to help improve power and increase clubhead speed. These workouts train the large muscles to "fire" in a similar explosive fashion used in the golf swing. If you are in good physical condition and are looking to improve your distance, consider adding a few explosive exercises to your fitness routine.

The following exercises have been designed for elite golfers to test their explosive power. The tests are designed to spot a possible power leak and help diagnose any major imbalances in your swing to locate where you are actually getting your power. According to the Titleist Performance Institute, the explosiveness needed to perform these tests is directly related to ball speed, precisely what is needed to hit the ball farther.[2]

THE GOLF POWER-SPECIFIC SCREEN

1. The Vertical Jump Test

This test measures the overall explosive power coming from your lower body. It is a good indication of how much explosiveness you have coming from your squat, lift, thrust, and bend movements, which are important for a powerful golf swing. The range for an elite player would be between 18 and 22 inches off the ground and between 25 and 28 inches for a typical long-drive Tour player.

HOW TO PERFORM THE TEST

- Standing against a wall, reach up as high as possible (while remaining flat-footed) with one arm and place a piece of tape on the wall.

- Jump as high as you can, placing another piece of tape at that level above the first piece.
- Repeat this exercise three to five times. Measure the difference in inches between the highest piece of tape and the first piece you placed on the wall.

Scoring Your Results
1 point   If the distance measures 15 inches or less.
2 points   If the distance measures 15 to 18 inches.
3 points   If the distance measures 18 inches or higher.

If you scored less than 2 points, consider working on the strength of and explosive power in your legs. If your legs are weak or much stronger than other parts of your body, it could lead to a number of swing flaws, including loss of balance, loss of width throughout the swing, and loss of posture.

2. The Medicine Ball Sit Up and Throw Test

This test measures the overall explosive power and strength in your core muscles and latissimus dorsi. The range of an elite player is 18 to 22 feet and 25 to 28 feet for a typical long-drive Tour player.

HOW TO PERFORM THE TEST

You will need a medicine ball for this test (five pounds for juniors and women, 10 pounds for men).

- Find a place where you can throw the ball 10 to 20 yards.
- Lie on your back with knees bent and feet flat on the ground and hold the medicine ball in both hands directly over your head as if you were going to toss a soccer ball.
- Sit up and throw the ball as far as possible.
- Repeat this process three times, and have a friend measure from your chest (sitting up) to the spot where the ball bounces on the floor.

Scoring Your Results
1 point   If the distance measures 15 feet or less.
2 points   If the distance measures 15 to 18 feet.
3 points   If the distance measures 18 feet or longer.

If you scored less than 2 points, consider working on the strength in your core and back muscles. Lack of power in the core can result in a number of swing flaws, including limited torso rotation, loss of spine angle, and power loss on the downswing.

3. Seated Chest Pass Test

This test measures the explosive power from your upper body, specifically your chest and triceps. The range for an elite player is between 18 to 22 feet and 25 to 28 feet for a typical long-drive Tour player.

HOW TO PERFORM THE TEST

- Get a medicine ball (five pounds for juniors and women, 10 pounds for men).
- Sit in a chair with your back pressed against the back of the chair.
- Hold the medicine ball against your chest and throw it as far as possible without letting your back come away from the back of the chair.
- Repeat the exercise three times, and have a friend measure the spot from your chest to where the ball bounces on the floor.

Scoring Your Results

1 point	If the distance measures 15 feet or less.
2 points	If the distance measures 15 to 18 feet.
3 points	If the distance measures 18 feet or longer.

If you scored 2 or less points, consider working to increase the strength and power in your upper body. If your upper body is weak or stronger than other parts of your body, it can lead to several swing flaws, including reverse pivot, loss of posture, and early release at impact.

Scoring

Vertical Jump Test Score	_____
Medicine Ball Sit Up and Throw Test Score	_____
Seated Chest Pass Test Score	_____
Total Score	_____/9

Evaluating Your Results

8–9 POINTS: OPTIMAL GOLF POWER SPECIFIC RATING

Congratulations, you passed the golf-specific power screen. Continue to maintain your fitness level. Remember that flexibility and strength decline with age, so work to maintain this level of fitness by doing the exercises and drills from this book. There should be no physical reason that your swing and game cannot improve. Assess your swing mechanics, scoring statistics, and mental attitude to determine which areas of your game to work on to improve your score. If you scored less than 2 points in any one area of the test, pay special attention to that area of the body.

6–7 POINTS: AVERAGE GOLF POWER SPECIFIC RATING

Your explosive power fitness level may need some improvement. Striving to improve your power and speed will not only help you gain club-head speed, but greater strength will help you prevent injuries. There may be a physical limitation that is holding you back from playing your best golf. Consider improving your fitness level through a proper training program like the one advised in this book. If you scored less than 2 points in any one area of the test, pay special attention to that area of the body.

5 POINTS OR LESS: BELOW GOLF POWER SPECIFIC RATING

Do not be discouraged. Although you may not be as fit as you could be, you could see a considerable amount of improvement in your golf game just by adding a few golf-specific exercises. You can overcome your physical limitations by beginning a fitness program to improve your strength and flexibility like the one advised in this book. If you scored less than 2 points in any one area of the test, pay special attention to those areas of the body.

REASONS TO PERFORM A BASIC GOLF-SPECIFIC FITNESS SCREEN

- to determine your strengths and weaknesses so you can develop a proper golf-specific fitness program based on your needs
- to detect physical problems so that you can improve functional fitness and athletic performance
- to create a functional baseline to mark your progress
- to determine if you have symmetrical limitations (both sides of the body) or asymmetrical limitations (one side of the body)
- to reduce the potential for training and sports injuries
- to determine your stability, or the ability to hold yourself in a certain position for a period of time
- to provide a simple grading system to assess your movement patterns
- to determine your strength, flexibility, and mobility

CHAPTER 4

WARM-UP 101

Essentials to Better Play and Minimizing Risk of Injury

THE KEY TO BETTER PLAY AND MINIMIZING RISK OF INJURY

Studies show that 53 percent of amateur golfers and 30 percent of professional golfers have sustained an injury while playing golf, and most of those injuries occurred while hitting balls on the golf course and practicing on the driving range. Professional golfers have more overuse injuries due to hours of practice, while weekend golfers are more likely to get injured from lack of conditioning and poor swing mechanics. While you may not think of the golf course as being hazardous to your health, there is the potential risk of suffering serious injuries to the wrists, elbows, lower back, hips, and knees while playing golf. Warming up is the easiest and most effective way to prevent injuries that can occur during practice and play.

If you have ever participated in a sport or some form of exercise, you have likely performed some type of regular warm-up and cool down before and after competition. So why wouldn't you warm up before a round of golf or a practice session? Swinging a golf club up to 300 times a round, including practice swings, at speeds upward of 90 miles per hour stresses our muscles, tendons, and joints to their full capacity.

Injury rates for recreational golfers are at an astounding 50 percent, and this number goes even higher for golfers over age 50. Recreational golfers have typically skipped warming up before play and practice because of the misconception that golf is not a strenuous activity, or due to time constraints. We are all so busy that when we have time to play golf we are anxious to get out on the golf course, and end up skipping the warm-up. But skipping the warm-up may mean that it takes us four or five holes before we loosen up and gain our form, and by that time our score may already have suffered. A few minutes warming up before the first tee can help you not only avoid those big numbers on your scorecard the first few holes but also prevent injury.

Professional golfers now know that a proper warm-up is essential for peak performance. Most recreational golfers haven't quite caught on to the trend, as they typically go straight from their car to the first tee and wonder why they don't hit a solid shot until the fifth or sixth hole. No matter what level of player you are, a proper warm-up can help you play your best golf and prevent injuries.

What does "warming up" mean? What types of warm-ups are best for golfers? How long should a warm-up last? Is stretching the same as warming up? Do you need special equipment to perform a warm-up? This chapter addresses these questions and provides a variety of warm-up routines for use throughout the year before play and practice.

WARMING UP

Warming up is the process of increasing muscle temperature, which in turn increases blood flow to bring needed oxygen to the muscles and joints. Warming up helps loosen stiff muscles and joints, making it easier for you to swing the golf club more efficiently. There are two ways to warm up: actively and passively. Active warm-ups (also called dynamic warm-ups) are achieved by any physical activity involving the large muscles of the body, mainly the torso, arms, and legs. Passive warm-ups can be accomplished by sitting in a steam room or taking a hot bath or shower. A golf-specific warm-up should include motions using the specific muscles utilized in the golf swing, as well as motions mimicking the swing itself.

THE BENEFITS OF WARMING UP

Warming up your body before practicing or playing a round of golf can greatly impact your golf swing and performance on the course. There are numerous physiological and psychological benefits to warming up, according to John Hinds, a physical therapist specializing in golf conditioning. Hinds says that a warm-up prepares the body for activity by promoting more efficient movement patterns through increased flexibility and blood flow. Hinds goes on to articulate that a proper warm-up helps tune the neuromuscular system, optimizing muscle force production (strength and power) and coordination and reinforcing proper movement patterns specific to the golf swing. Sufficient preparation also reduces the risk of injury.

A golf-specific warm-up also does the following:

- improves range of motion to help you make a complete shoulder turn and follow-through
- prepares golf-specific muscles to move more efficiently
- increases blood flow to loosen and relax stiff muscles
- increases energy
- decreases lactic acid buildup in muscles so you won't be sore after your round
- provides a rehearsal for movements that you will be performing throughout the day
- allows you time to prepare your mind for concentrating on your golf game for four to five hours
- reduces the chance of injury
- increases physical capacity
- elevates energy levels
- raises resistance to fatigue
- improves mental awareness and cognitive function
- decreases anxiety
- enhances performance

HOW TO WARM UP BEFORE PLAY OR PRACTICE

According to the *Journal of Strength and Conditioning Research*, those who warm up specifically for their sport perform better than those who do not. Most people think that static stretching is the correct way to warm up before a round of golf, and while stretching is advisable, you actually need to warm up before you stretch. You should incorporate an active warm-up specifically for golf before you stretch. An active warm-up incorporates the large muscles of the upper body and lower body and requires you to move at a brisk pace for 5 to 10 minutes to elevate your heart rate.

For younger players, the goal is to break a sweat. For older golfers, the objective is to become slightly winded. Activities that raise your heart rate include walking, jogging, doing jumping jacks, or even something as simple as swinging two clubs back and forth. These types of movements gradually warm up the cardiovascular and muscular systems. An active warm-up should always be performed prior to stretching.

Once you have completed an active warm-up, you are ready to move into the golf-specific phase of the warm-up, also known as movement rehearsal. During this phase, we are literally rehearsing the moves required to execute the golf swing.

The following is a review of how to warm up prior to a practice round or round of golf:

- Warm up first, no matter how long you are going to play or practice.
- Do an active warm-up for 5 to 10 minutes by doing some sort of physical activity, like walking or jogging, to get your heart rate elevated and blood circulating. If your facility has a gym, get on a treadmill or stationary bike for a few minutes. Jogging, doing jumping jacks, or simply walking briskly will also do the trick.
- Follow the active warm-up with 5 to 10 minutes of golf-specific movements and stretches to rehearse the golf swing. You will find several examples of golf-specific stretches in this book.

The subsequent sections provide a variety of warm-up tips and routines designed by our GFM team for use year-round. The routines will take you anywhere from 2 minutes to 30 minutes to complete and include a balanced combination of rhythmic limbering exercises and dynamic and static stretches for the entire body. Doing a warm-up before you play or practice is the most important factor in the success and enjoyment of your next round of golf. Find something that works for your routine, time, and facility constraints. Consult a golf fitness professional who can design a warm-up routine that will help you play your best golf.

WARM UP LIKE THE PROS

Almost every professional on Tour today performs a preround warm-up routine prior to teeing it up, according to Sean Cochran, one of the most recognized golf fitness trainers in the world today. He travels the PGA Tour regularly working with PGA professionals, most notably two-time Masters and PGA champion Phil Mickelson. The routines he has his players do prepare them for the upcoming round mentally, physically, and biomechanically. This preparation is an integral part of success during a round.

The goals of a warm-up program are numerous, and as a result, such a program has positive effects on a round of golf. By looking at the format of a PGA Tour player's warm-up routine, we can learn a lot about how to develop our own program. As weekend or occasional golfers, we do not necessarily have the prep time prior to a round that exists for the professional player, but if we utilize the same structure, incorporate the correct exercises and drills, and spend our time wisely, we can acquire the same benefits as the professionals in as little as 15 minutes. In addition to preparing the body to swing a club, such exercises assist in preparing your mind to focus on the task ahead. The following is a sample preround warm-up program used by many PGA Tour professionals. Program guidelines are as follows:

- Perform a single set of each exercise.
- Complete 10 to 15 repetitions of each exercise.
- Perform each exercise to the best of your ability.
- Remember to not overdo it. This is just a warm-up.

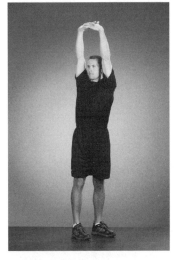

FIGURE 4.1

Tops

Goal: Increase the range of motion in the shoulder capsules and core.

- Begin with the arms straight overhead, fingers clasped together, and feet shoulder-width apart (see figure 4.1).
- Rotate the hips to the left and then to the right, pausing for one second at the end point of each rotation.
- Repeat the rotation back and forth for 10 to 15 repetitions.

Windmills

Goal: Loosen up the lower and upper back.

- Rotate your arms and shoulders as far to the left as possible, keeping the heels on the ground (see figure 4.2). Pause for one second.
- Rotate as far to the right as possible. Pause for one second.
- Perform 10 to 15 rotations left and right.

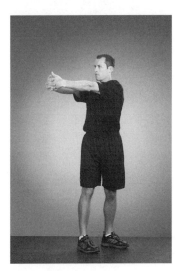

FIGURE 4.2

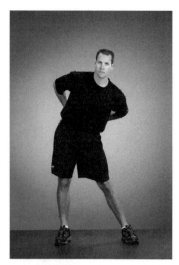

FIGURE 4.3

Hip Circles

Goal: Increase the range of motion in the hips and lower back.

- Stand with your feet slightly wider than shoulder-width apart, hands in the small of the lower back, and eyes looking forward. Slowly rotate the hips in a large circle to your left. Allow your hips, knees, and ankles to rotate (see figure 4.3).
- Perform 10 to 15 repetitions to your left, and repeat in the opposite direction.

Rotators

Goal: Warm up the hamstrings and lower back.

- Place the feet shoulder-width apart, arms extended overhead, hands clasped together, and eyes looking forward.
- Rotate the torso, shoulders, arms, and head to the right.
- Extend your hands downward to the outside of the right foot. Pause for one second.
- Extend downward to the level where you can feel the stretch in either the hamstrings or lower back (see figure 4.4).
- Return to the starting position.
- Repeat the same sequence to the left. Perform 10 to 15 repetitions.

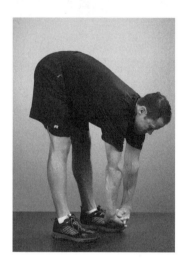

FIGURE 4.4

PREROUND WARM-UP ROUTINES

One of the goals at GFM is to encourage our readers to emulate the professionals by getting into the habit of performing preround warm-up routines on a regular basis. Most golf fitness professionals, like David Donatucci, the director of fitness and performance at the PGA Learning Center at the PGA Golf Club, located in Port St. Lucie, Florida, agree that warming up is the key to playing your best golf.

The team at GFM asked Donatucci to show golfers a warm-up routine that doesn't take too much time. Donatucci says that the ideal warm-up should be a series of dynamic stretches that mimic the motions used in the golf swing and involve all of the major muscles. His entire routine takes only two minutes, so there's no excuse not to warm up before you play.

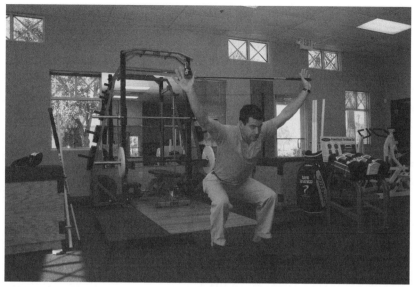

FIGURE 4.5

Deep Overhead Squats

- Assume your golf address position.
- Raise a golf club over your head with arms extended.
- Slowly squat down as low as you can as you maintain the club above your head (see figure 4.5).
- Return to the starting position.
- Do six to eight repetitions.

Shoulder Rotations

- Assume your golf address position.
- Grip a club so that it is parallel to the ground with your palms facing downward.
- Slowly raise the club above and behind your head (see figure 4.6).
- Return to the starting position.
- Do six to eight repetitions.

Hip Rotations

- Turn a club upside down and use it for balance.
- Stand on one leg.

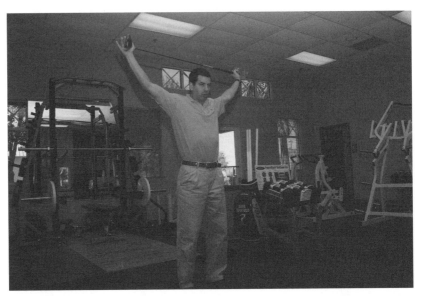

FIGURE 4.6

- Rotate the hip from side to side as you maintain your shoulders square (see figure 4.7).
- Rotate the hip back and forth for six to eight repetitions.
- Return to the starting position and repeat the exercise on the other leg.

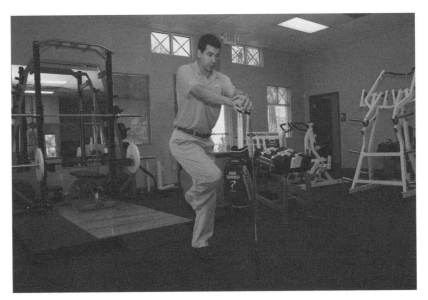

FIGURE 4.7

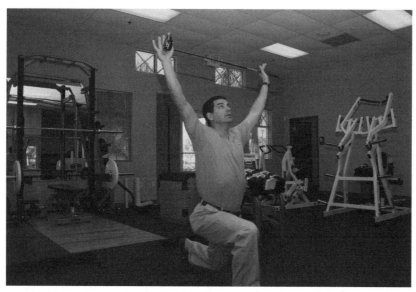

FIGURE 4.8

Lunges with Back Extensions

- Stand with your feet shoulder-width apart and grip a club so that it is parallel with the ground.
- Step forward with one leg and drop your knee so that it forms a 90-degree angle.
- Lift the club above your head, and look up to the sky (see figure 4.8).
- Return to the starting position.
- Repeat the exercise with the opposite leg.
- Alternate lunges for six to eight repetitions.

Single-Leg Balances with Rotations

- Assume your golf address position.
- Place a club across your chest.
- Lift one leg.
- Rotate your shoulders to the right and left (see figure 4.9).
- Rotate your shoulders for six to eight repetitions.
- Repeat the exercise with the opposite leg.

When you have completed this routine, take a few practice swings, and you are warmed up and ready to play.

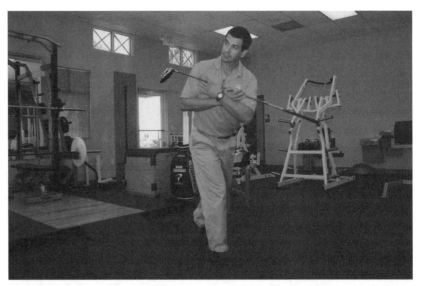

FIGURE 4.9

MAKE OVER YOUR WARM-UP

Many people think stretching is a way to warm up before golf, because, if you are like most of us, you were taught the importance of warm-up calisthenics back in grade school and have pretty much stuck with the same routine ever since. Exercise science, however, has moved on. Researchers now believe that regular stretching is not only a waste of time, but also bad for you. Holding a static stretch for 20 to 30 seconds can weaken your muscles if you have not properly prepared them. You should actually warm up muscles, tendons, and joints *before* your stretch. In essence, you need to warm up before your warm up.

To update your warm-up routine, follow this sequence: First, raise your body temperature to increase your blood flow, which brings needed oxygen to muscles, tendons, and joints. Second, only after muscles are warm, do stretches to increase your range of motion in muscles that mimic the movements you are going to be doing for the rest of the day.

To raise your body's temperature, a warm-up should begin with an aerobic activity, for example, walking, knee raises, jogging in place, or jumping jacks. For younger players, the goal is to break a sweat; for older golfers it is to become slightly winded. The aerobic portion of your warm-up should take only two to three minutes, just enough time to warm up your body.

For stretching to be beneficial to your game, you should simulate the golf swing as much as possible. Doing stretches that mimic the golf swing will prepare the muscles for the motions that you will be doing for the next four to five hours.

WARMING UP IN HOT WEATHER

It may seem counterintuitive to stretch and warm up before a round of golf when it is hot outside because you may already be sweating, but it is just as important to perform your preround warm-up routine in hot weather as it is in cold weather. "Stretching or a pregolf warm-up should be done regardless of temperature," says Andrea Doddato, founder of Shape and Sport in Orlando, Florida. Golf performance coach Dave Herman, whose clients include Trevor Immelman and Suzann Pettersen, agrees. He states that "muscles and joints like warm weather, and they tend to respond more quickly to heat, so warm-up exercises are always beneficial to your golf game in hot and cold weather."

Warming up your body in the summer heat is different than warming up your body in cold weather. There are a few things that you should do differently and precautions you should take. "In hot weather, a player should really only focus on chronically tight areas," says Doddato. "Say the golfer is hyper-mobile (too loose) within his shoulder girdle. In cold weather, stretching the shoulder would not negatively impact this joint, but in hot weather, when the body temperature heats up beyond normal, the joint becomes too elastic and can be more prone to injury. The player almost wants to keep the joint a bit tighter." You may not have to stretch as much as you do in colder weather.

Another thing to take into consideration while warming up in the heat is that your body temperature will rise more quickly when you initiate physical activity. Normally, a person who exercises and is in good condition can handle temperature ranges of 65 to 85 degrees Fahrenheit, but as the temperature rises, special precautions need to be taken. "In hot weather, it can be wise to warm up indoors so you have less fluid loss before the round," says Herman.

The following are a few hot-weather tips to make your preround warm-up routine safe and effective during warmer weather:

1. *Stay hydrated*. Drink 8 ounces of water 30 minutes prior to starting your warm-up routine. During your round, drink 3 to 6 ounces of water every 20 minutes or every 2 holes. After your round, drink 8 ounces of water within 30 minutes of playing the last hole.

2. *Lower intensity levels*. When warming up in the heat, you don't have to work as hard to elevate your heart rate.

3. *Avoid playing and practicing during the hottest times of the day*. Take advantage of the extra daylight. Early morning and evening hours allow for cooler temperatures to get in a round of golf.

4. *Keep your warm-up routine indoors*. Perform your warm-up routine in the house before you leave for the day or do it in

the locker room. An air-conditioned environment provides total protection from the heat. If you must do your routine outside, perform it in the shade.

5. *Adjust clothing.* Wear lightweight, loose fitting, and light colored clothes. Don't skip the socks. Light cotton socks will protect the feet and help wick sweat away. Warm up before your round of golf regardless of the weather. A proper warm-up will get your muscles accustomed to increased activity and reduce the risk of stiffness later.

. . . .

■ Ladies Tee
RETHINK YOUR PREROUND ROUTINE

What does your warm-up routine look like before you make your first swing of the day? Do you get out of your car, drive a cart to the range, do a couple of static stretches, and think you are good to go? This type of warm-up has been around for so long it is ingrained in almost every golfer's head, as if to imply it is the only way to get ready to play. What golfers don't realize is that the golf swing is a violent, unnatural movement that requires a high degree of coordination. Doing static stretches before you play has no benefit and could even harm you if you stretch "cold" ligaments and tendons.

Unfortunately, with the time constraints of motherhood and full-time jobs, the last thing women think of is warming up before a round of golf. But spending time preparing to play can not only increase the body's core temperature, loosening up muscles and making them more elastic, supple, and pliable so it is easier to swing, it can also help prevent injuries.

Because of their low-efficiency movements, most high-handicap players spend up to 95 percent of their total energy output on a swing, with poor results. A dynamic warm-up will not only "wake up" the body's nervous system, but also prepare it for the high-demand movements required to make it more efficient, so you don't have to work so hard to execute a good swing. If you have been accepting the "norm" of static stretching before you play, it is time to rethink your preround routine.

A proper warm-up does not need to take a tremendous amount of time. Four to five minutes will do the trick. It will not only loosen your body up to help you swing more efficiently, but this routine will get you into a good frame of mind to start your round out right. Adopt the following as your preround warm-up routine to better your golf game:

1. *Jumping rope.* Jumping rope can be done anywhere and is an excellent way to warm up the entire body within a few minutes. It will also stimulate your nervous system, the connection between your mind, hands, and feet. Jump rope for one to three minutes. See figure 4.10.

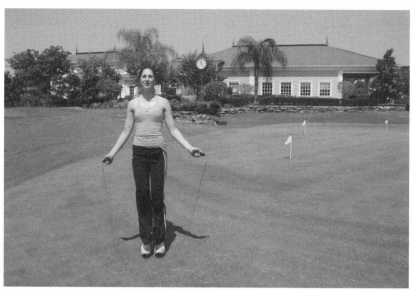

FIGURE 4.10

2. *Jumping jacks*. Jumping jacks are also an efficient way to warm up the body. Performing jumping jacks requires coordination, helping hone your motor skills. Perform 10 to 15 repetitions. See figure 4.11.

3. *Shoulder rotations*. Simple shoulder rotations will help you warm up your body and increase your shoulder turn in the golf swing. Keeping your arms and shoulders relaxed, engage your core muscles as you rotate. Minimize lateral movement by imagining that you are rotating inside of a cylinder. Do 12 to 15 repetitions. See figure 4.12.

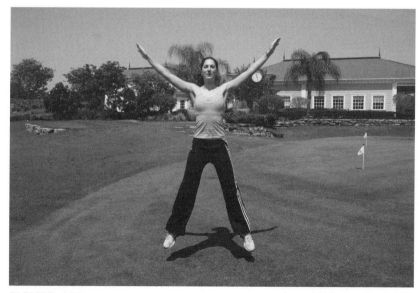

FIGURE 4.11

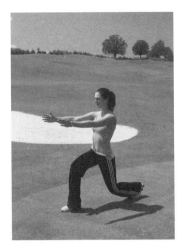

FIGURE 4.13

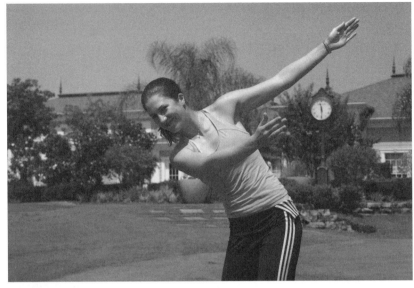

FIGURE 4.12

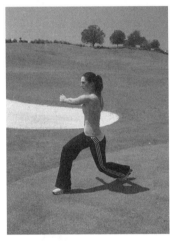

FIGURE 4.14

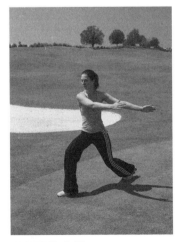

FIGURE 4.15

4. *Standing lunges with rotation*. Performing standing lunges with rotation will wake up your gluteal muscles, test your balance, and warm up your spine. Maintain a relaxed upper body as you engage your core muscles. Keep your front knee bent at a 90-degree angle. Perform 6 to 8 rotations for each leg. See figures 4.13, 4.14, and 4.15.

5. *Push-ups*. Push-ups, although not typically thought of as a warm-up exercise, are great for creating a solid connection between your hands and feet, enabling you to create a concrete foundation for your swing. Use your abdominal muscles to pull the body up into position as you push up. Perform 6 to 10 repetitions.

PUTTING IT ALL TOGETHER

We have shown you a variety of warm-up exercises to help prepare for both play and practice. But how do you know which exercises are the best for warming up before play? It is important to do a variety of exercises and stretches that target different parts of the body. You may find that one specific routine suits your needs, so stick with that one, just make sure that it includes an active warm-up to loosen muscles and golf-specific stretches. If you like, you can mix it up and do a different routine each time you play. The important thing is that you are performing some sort of preround warm-up each time you play. The following is an example of a preround routine that contains all the key elements of a proper warm-up.

1. *Walk to the driving range or first tee to get the blood pumping and flowing to your muscles.* "Even if I only have five minutes, I walk around the driving range or hop on the treadmill (there is one in the locker room at my club). This simple act warms up my legs, back, and upper body. I even try to work up a sweat," says Art Sellinger, two-time Long Drive Championship winner.

2. *Hit five balls without rushing through them.* Instead of indiscriminately firing off one shot after another, trying to finish off an entire bucket before you play, hit only a few balls with a mid-iron and take more time. This will help relax you, and you won't feel rushed as you get to the first tee. Do a golf-specific stretch in between each shot. Put the club behind your back and make a backswing swing and hold the position for a few moments. Try to increase your shoulder turn with each shot. Pick one of the exercises or stretches that we have shown you in this chapter.

3. *Hit four putts different distances.* Take four balls to the putting green before you tee off (there is usually a practice green next to the first tee) and putt balls to different targets to get your feel. Finish with a few two-foot putts to hear the ball go in the cup for confidence and head to the first tee.

SUMMARY

A proper warm-up is essential for peak performance in golf. Tour professionals know the benefits of warming up and have incorporated routines into both practice and play. Although recreational golfers may not have the time or equipment available to professional golfers, they can still do simple exercises like those demonstrated in this chapter to prepare themselves for playing their best. Warming up is the easiest and most effective way to prevent injuries during practice and play.

CHAPTER 5

SHAPE YOUR GAME

Strength, flexibility, coordination, and balance will help golfers at all levels play their best golf. Choosing which exercises to do to change your swing faults and strengthen your weaknesses are the key to dramatically improving your game; however, with a number of exercises and routines to choose from and such compounding factors as lack of time and money, there are a few things to consider, including the following:

1. *Effective routines are those that you can easily perform and stick with for an extended period of time.* Avoid complicated, time consuming routines. Golf fitness is about finding the right balance of exercise, practice, and play. You can dramatically improve your game with just a few exercises per day. There is no need to spend hours in the gym.

2. *Choose routines that can be performed in your home or a gym where you are already a member.* There is no need to join expensive specialized gyms or buy bulky, expensive equipment. Most of the golf-specific routines demonstrated in this book can be done with minimal equipment and in the comfort of your own home.

3. *Choose routines that are safe and effective for your particular needs.* Avoid unsafe exercises and routines that will make you so sore that you abandon them after only a few days. Golf fitness is a lifestyle, and you will want to choose exercises that not only help your golf game but keep you in shape and healthy for life.

According to GFM advisor Donald Wallace, who specializes in spinal rehabilitation and ectrodiagnostic studies, Vladimir Janda, the renowned neurologist and physical therapist, determined that there are certain muscles in our body that are prone to be weak and certain muscles that tend to be tight. Wallace notes that, interestingly enough, the muscles that tend to be weak and tight are the same muscles necessary for an elite golf swing. These weak or inhibited muscles need to be activated and strengthened to enable you to perform a biomechanically correct golf swing. The golf muscles that tend to be weak are the abdominal, hip, buttock, and lower back muscles. The muscles that tend to be tight are the inner thigh, hip, hamstring, and middle and lower back muscles. You should strive to do a variety of golf-specific routines that balance strength exercises with flexibility exercises for a complete golf-specific fitness program.

In chapter 1, we outlined the eight common swing faults and how to screen for physical limitations. In this chapter, we will demonstrate a few specific corrective exercises for you to use to counteract your swing faults and give you simple yet effective routines designed by our GFM team to help you shape your body to improve your game. These routines will help give you direction on how to begin to train for golf.

There are three keys to a complete golf fitness program: posture/balance, strength, and flexibility. Whether you are a seasoned athlete or just starting a golf fitness program, you will want to start by improving your posture and balance. Then move into doing resistance training to strengthen weak muscles. Last, you will want to work on your flexibility to increase and maintain your optimal range of motion.

You will find several golf-specific routines in this chapter that will help you stretch your golf muscles. These are only examples of exercises that can help you improve your golf fitness levels. They are by no means meant to be a stand-alone program but are to compliment other fitness programs that you may already follow. Consulting a golf fitness specialist or golf teacher certified in golf fitness who can evaluate your fitness level and design a golf-specific fitness program tailored to meet your needs is recommended.

POSTURE AND BALANCE

Before you dive headfirst into a full-blown golf fitness routine, pumping weights, and working on flexibility, it is first important to work on improving your posture, the base for any good golf swing. Creating symmetry within the body is essential to improving your swing. Strengthening opposing muscle groups is necessary to achieve this. In previous chapters, we took a look at how poor posture can inhibit the body from functioning properly. One of those poor posture scenarios is C-posture, a posture that occurs when the shoulders are slumped forward at address position and there is a definitive roundness in the back extending from the tailbone to the back of the neck. It is common in individuals who have poor or slumped posture. If a golfer has this type of posture, it will limit the extent to which the torso and shoulders are able to rotate on the backswing. The following sections detail a few key exercises that will help you develop this balance and correct C-posture. Stretches are also included to correct shortening of the shoulder muscles.

1. The External Rotator Cuff Exercise with Resistance Band

Three of the four rotator cuff muscles are found on the backside of the shoulder. These muscles are responsible for keeping the shoulder girdle in place. Risk of injury occurs when these muscles are weak or unbalanced because they are fighting to pull the shoulder joint back into alignment from its forward, rounded posture. The following exercise will help strengthen these three muscles:

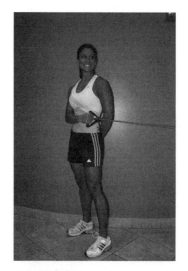

FIGURE 5.1

- Place a resistance band around a stable object and stand sideways, with one arm facing the object the band is wrapped around and one arm facing away from the object.
- Hold the free end of the resistance band in the hand farthest from the object.
- Keep the band at elbow level, holding your arm in a 90-degree angle.
- From the center of the body, rotate your arm away from the body, maintaining a 90-degree angle of the arm (see figures 5.1 and 5.2).
- Do 3 sets of 12 to 15 repetitions with each arm.

2. The Reverse Fly Exercise with Dumbbells

Not only do the external rotator cuff muscles need to be strengthened to help alleviate C-posture, but you also need to strengthen the large back portion of the shoulder. More often than not, this exercise is performed incorrectly, and only the muscles close to the shoulder blade are used.

- Get a pair of three- to five-pound dumbbells.
- Sit or stand (standing will incorporate the core and leg muscles that are used in the golf swing) and bend at the waist, forming as

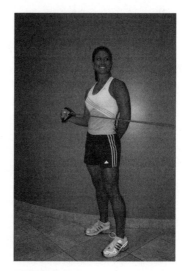

FIGURE 5.2

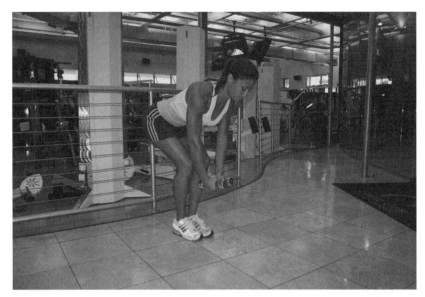

FIGURE 5.3

close to a 90-degree angle as possible with upper body and lower body.

- Start with your hands in front of you, and extend them in a straight line to the side until they are parallel with the floor. The weights should align with your head when your arms are fully extended. Don't let your arms droop (see figures 5.3 and 5.4).
- Do 3 sets of 12 to 15 repetitions every other day.

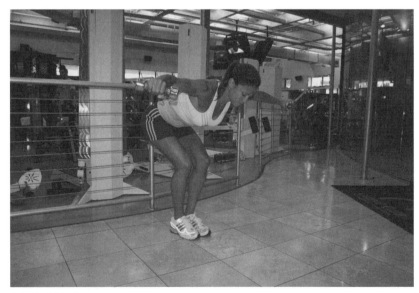

FIGURE 5.4

3. Bent-Over Dumbbell Rows

It is important to develop the muscles surrounding the back of the shoulder but also the muscles that surround the shoulder blade. One of the functions of these muscles is to retract, and with C-posture, the shoulder and shoulder blades are in a constant state of protraction. This exercise will help you correct this problem. The bent-over dumbbell row will also incorporate the core and leg muscles. This is beneficial in correcting C-posture and should be performed twice a week. Choose a weight that is challenging but doesn't hinder you from performing the exercise properly.

- Get a pair of three- to five-pound dumbbells.
- Standing next to a bench or stable object, bend at the waist, and fully extend one arm down toward the ground.
- Using the fully extended arm, pull the weight back and up, keeping the elbow close to your trunk. Limit the rotation of your trunk as you raise and lower the weight (see figures 5.5 and 5.6).
- Do 12 to 15 repetitions with each arm.

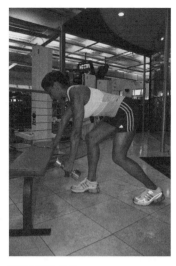

FIGURE 5.5

4. Seated Rows

Seated rows take the lower body out of the exercise and incorporate both arms. You will want to use a seated row machine for this exercise.

- Sit on the bench and extend your arms out in front of you, grabbing the weight with both hands.
- Pull the weight back in one motion, keeping your back straight and chest up.
- At the end of the motion, squeeze your shoulder blades together and then release weight forward (see figure 5.7 and 5.8).
- Do 12 to 15 repetitions.

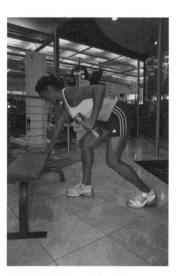

FIGURE 5.6

5. Stretching

Strengthening opposing muscle groups is necessary to correct C-posture, but you must also stretch the muscles that are causing the shortening that results in the rounding of the shoulder muscles. This shortening limits the tendency of these two opposing forces to work against each other. Two good stretches are the forward chest stretch and the behind the back stretch.

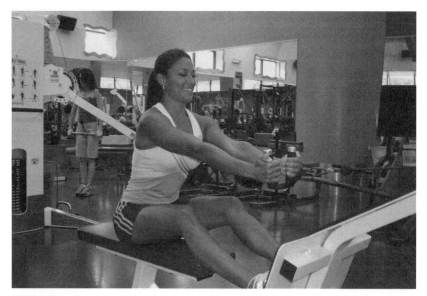

FIGURE 5.7

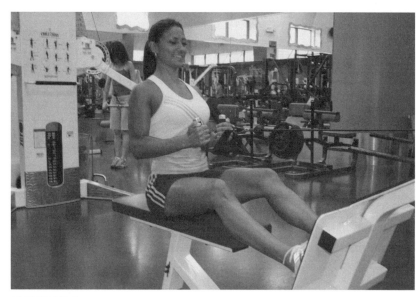

FIGURE 5.8

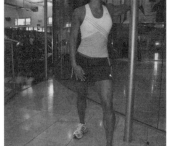

FIGURE 5.9

THE FORWARD CHEST STRETCH

- Find a doorway or pole.
- Place one arm on the door or pole at a 90-degree angle and step forward with the same leg (see figure 5.9).
- To increase the stretch and involve the upper portion of the chest, lean the upper body downward so that you are looking at the floor.
- Hold the position for 20 to 30 seconds.

THE BEHIND THE BACK STRETCH

- Place a towel or a golf club behind your head and grab the lower end with the other hand behind your back.
- Pull upward toward the head. You should feel a stretch in the front part of the shoulder. Be careful to not overstretch (see figure 5.10).
- Hold the position for 20 to 30 seconds.
- Repeat the stretch with the opposite arm.

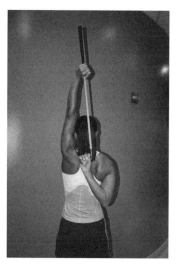

FIGURE 5.10

How to Work on Your Balance for a Better Swing

Long hitters get their distance and power from speed, and although they swing the club fast, they never lose their balance. When most high-handicappers try to get more distance, they swing the club too quickly and lose their balance. One of the most overlooked keys to power and distance is balance, which affects almost every phase of the swing. Having good balance helps your body turn and shift weight more effectively, assists your body in making a smooth transition from the backswing to the downswing, and allows your body to create more clubhead speed.

Balance is just like muscle strength in that you need to work at it or you will lose it. As we age, our sight, hearing, muscle strength, coordination, and reflexes change, weakening our balance. Such health conditions as diabetes, heart disease, and circulation problems can also affect balance. Improving your balance takes time and practice, and it doesn't just happen overnight; however, with practice, you should be able to improve your balance over time and see improvement in your golf swing. Incorporating balance exercises into your preround warm-up routine is a great way to improve your balance.

....

■ Ladies Tee
BALLET AND GOLF

The golf swing is a dance move in itself, similar to the moves in ballet. Both arts require a great deal of finesse, balance, coordination, flow, flexibility, and strength without bulky muscles, not to mention focus and concentration. Practicing ballet movements can be ideal for enhancing your prowess and enjoyment of the game, because ballet incorporates a range of motions similar to the movements of a golf swing. These moves coordinate into a beautiful form, creating a beautiful outcome. This is a workout you can't get on a treadmill.

LPGA (Ladies Professional Golf Association) Tour player Kris Tschetter took ballet classes as a child and then took them up again as an adult. According to Tschetter, "Taking ballet classes has helped me mentally on the golf course. When you are dancing, you are so focused inward on what you are doing that you are not aware of the distractions around you. The focus I have learned from ballet is what has helped me most in golf."

Ballet can improve your golf game in the following ways:

- *Builds leg strength*. Ballet will strengthen your legs to help create a more powerful swing.
- *Develops focus*. Ballet can help improve your focus. To properly execute ballet moves, you must be able to focus and ignore distractions while you learn to use different muscle groups and body parts.
- *Fosters core strength*. The center of movement in the body is your core, which includes your back, abdominal, and hamstring muscles, and ballet is another way to strengthen the core area. A strong core is an integral part of preventing back injuries.

Attention guys: Real men do ballet. Ballet can be extremely beneficial for men. Football players have been using ballet for years as a way to create better flexibility and coordination on the football field. Since almost every muscle is used in ballet, it helps build the flexibility that may be lacking in your golf swing, and muscle movements become more flowing. The muscles used in executing the golf swing are at their best when they are long, lean, and fast, not bulky and slow.

....

STRENGTH

To create power and speed in your golf swing, it is important to strengthen weak muscles. Many golfers are reluctant to lift weights in fear of developing big muscles, therefore losing feel and flexibility. Resistance training specific for golf will not result in muscle gain that will alter your swing mechanics.

Increasing muscle size, the way body builders do, involves lifting increasingly heavier weights with lower repetitions, increasing your calorie intake dramatically, and spending many hours per day lifting weights.

A golf-specific fitness program incorporates moderate weight lifting with medium (12 to 15) repetitions for 30 to 40 minutes two to three times per week. This type of program is designed to improve your golf-specific strength and endurance, not build muscle.

If you are just beginning a golf-specific training program, start out by using light weights and small amounts of resistance. As you become stronger, you can add resistance and heavier weights to gain more power. By strengthening the muscles specific to golf, you will have better control of your body. When you improve functional strength, you have more control and balance, which will improve your feel. The strength training routines presented here will help you not only gain muscular control and coordination, but also more power and endurance.

Strengthen Your Core for Better Golf

Most fitness professionals agree that your "core," or torso (made up of the abdominal, back, hip, and chest muscles), is essentially the "engine of the body." It is the area of the body that initiates most human movement, including the golf swing. A strong, flexible core allows you to turn your trunk to create power and speed. If your core is weak and inflexible, it is difficult to swing the club with power and stay balanced. Since your core must rotate in both directions during the golf swing, it is important to perform rotational exercises that develop both strength and flexibility.

Golf-Specific Fitness for Women

The muscles of the core may be the most important golf muscles used to create power and speed in your swing, but your forearms, hands, and wrists square the clubface for consistency. Your hands are your only connection to the golf club, and they control the direction in which the ball flies. Women typically lack upper body strength, so the repetitive motions of golf and the high speed of the typical swing can place the wrists and hands at high risk for injury.

Pain and tenderness on top of the wrist experienced at the top of the backswing and at impact are common. The most frequent golf-related wrist injuries are tendinitis, or swelling of the tendons responsible for wrist movement, and bursitis. Both can occur in the hands, wrists, and elbows. If a player lacks strength in the hands, wrists, and forearms, he or she is more likely to sustain an injury through traumatic force resulting from a poorly executed golf swing, hitting a root or rock or taking a deep divot, and from overuse. The best way to prevent injury and improve your swing is to strengthen your hands and wrists.

Strength for a Better Short Game

It is well-documented that improving strength and flexibility helps you prevent injuries and gain more distance with your swing, but golf fitness experts have recently come to realize that fitness can also improve touch and finesse around the greens. The short game does not typically

HATE THE SAND, GET STRONGER

You will often hear television announcers say that professional golfers would rather hit out of the sand than out of the rough when they miss a green. That is because professionals have a better chance of getting the ball to spin out of the bunker than from the rough and are therefore able to get the ball to land softer and closer to the hole. Most high-handicappers hate the sand, likely because of a combination of bad technique and lack of hand and wrist strength to be used in getting themselves out.

First, the sand wedge is the heaviest club in the bag, thus a tremendous amount of hand and wrist strength is required to swing it. Second, in the sand you actually want to hit the sand first to explode the ball out of the bunker, so you need to swing the club at a high rate of speed to move the clubhead through the sand. If you are not strong enough, you will end up decelerating the clubhead at the moment of impact, and you will not be able to propel the ball out of the bunker. Developing hand and wrist strength will increase your chances of getting out of the bunker every single time with ease.

require the power associated with tee shots, but rather skill to control the distance the ball rolls on the green. Mastering the short game comes from motor control, and controlling your muscles and nerves and increasing motor control can come from improved fitness.

Unlike your long game, where a large portion of the power is generated through the core and legs, your short game requires fitness of an entirely different set of muscles. The muscles in the shoulders, arms, wrists, and hands initiate putts and wedge shots. Hinging the wrists correctly and setting the clubface in the correct position is imperative in hitting crisp chips and pitch shots. Accelerating through the sand is essential to getting out of bunkers. To perform these shots, a certain level of strength is needed in the upper body, so if the muscles within the shoulders, arms, wrists, and hands are weak and inflexible, you will not be able to create the shots you want around the green. Developing strength in the upper body is the easiest and fastest way to improve your short game.

FLEXIBILITY

Flexibility is the ability of the body to bend without breaking. It is what makes the body pliable. It is flexibility that allows the joints to bend repeatedly without injury. If you don't think this is important, think again, especially if you have noticed that it isn't quite as easy to turn your neck to look over your shoulder as you back out of the driveway, or if you have seen that your golf swing keeps getting shorter every year, as does the distance the ball flies off the tee. Flexibility allows you to make a complete shoulder turn in your backswing without bending your arms; it allows you to shift your weight smoothly on the downswing and follow-through on the finish. Flexibility is one of the most important elements of golf fitness.

Flexibility is limited by such factors as genetics, age, and lack of stretching. As we age, the tissues around our joints tend to thicken, so we lose range of motion in our joints and ligaments. But older people are not the only ones who need to worry about inflexibility. Flexibility also decreases as a result of inactivity, meaning that you will stiffen up if you don't work at staying flexible.

The good news is that studies show improvements in flexibility when individuals engage in exercise programs that involve stretching exercises. If you stretch your muscles, ligaments, and joints regularly, you may be able to prevent them from getting tighter and more restricted. Stretching is one of the easiest and fastest ways to improve your golf swing and game. Stretching will not only improve your flexibility to increase your range of motion in your muscles and joints to help you make a better shoulder turn, but when done on a daily basis, it can help improve your balance, prevent injuries, increase your circulation, and improve your muscle coordination.

Stretching does not require equipment or a change of clothes. Stretching habits can be slowly worked into a multitasking routine. Instead of sitting still while watching television or talking on the phone, stand up and perform a few golf-specific stretches. Commit to doing a few stretches before and after you play. Doing spontaneous stretching throughout the day for a minute or two can also help. Even if you only stretch for two to three minutes a day a few times a week, you will feel the difference in no time.

The following are a few basic golf-specific movements that will stretch your golf muscles. Incorporate them into your daily routine to improve your flexibility and your golf swing.

A TIP FOR STRETCHING IT OUT

Warm up your body first by walking around and pumping your arms to get blood and oxygen to muscles. Stretching "cold" muscles increases the risk of injury.

The Chest Opener on a Ball

- Get an exercise ball.
- Sit on the ball and place your hands behind your head, interlock your fingers, and lightly rest your head in your hands.
- Slowly walk your feet forward as the ball rolls under your upper back and neck until your knees are at a 90-degree angle. Keep the head and neck supported, engage the gluteal muscles, and maintain the hips parallel with the floor (see figures 5.11 and 5.12).
- Hold the stretch for 10 to 15 seconds. Focus on the stretch in the chest.
- Place your hands back on the ball, and walk your feet back to the starting position.

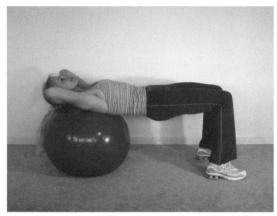

FIGURE 5.11

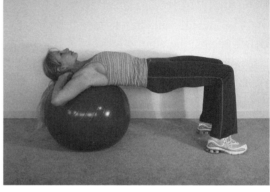

FIGURE 5.12

The Cat/Cow Pose

- Kneel on the floor on your hands and knees.
- Place your hands directly under your shoulders and knees directly under your hips.
- Inhale as you press your spine toward the floor, roll the shoulders back. Be sure not to hyperextend your neck (see figure 5.13).
- Exhale as you press your navel toward your spine, engage your gluteal muscles, press your spine toward the ceiling, and tuck the chin into the chest (see figure 5.14).
- Repeat this pose 10 times in each direction.

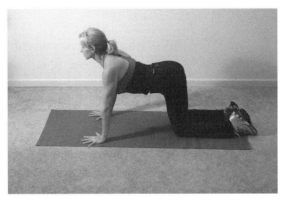

FIGURE 5.13

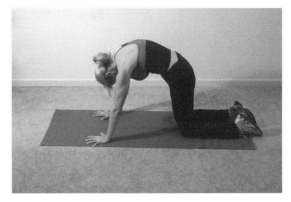

FIGURE 5.14

The Modified Cobra to Upward-Facing Dog

- Lie on the floor with your chest facing downward, palms placed below your shoulders, and elbows pressed against your body (see figure 5.15).
- Bring the legs together, squeeze your gluteal muscles, and, upon exhalation, lift your chest off of the floor (see figure 5.15).
- Roll the shoulders back away from your ears. Be sure not to hyperextend your neck.
- Return to the starting position and repeat five times.

The Upward-Facing Dog

- If you feel you are ready to move deeper into the stretch, roll to the tops of the feet and lift the legs off of the floor (see figure 5.16).
- Hold for three to five counts.

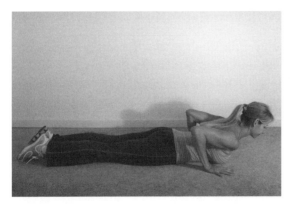

FIGURE 5.15

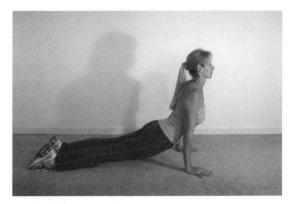

FIGURE 5.16

The Basic Bridge

This exercise challenges the stability of the pelvis, lower back, and core while strengthening your gluteal muscles. There are several variations of this exercise.

- Lie on your back with your knees bent and feet hip-distance apart.
- Focus on recruiting your gluteal muscles throughout the exercise rather than your hamstrings. This will take practice and concentration.
- Inhale as you begin and exhale as you lift your hips into a bridge position. Imagine a straight line from your shoulders to your knees (see figure 5.17).
- Inhale as you hold this position, and exhale as you lift one leg slightly off of the floor without shifting or dropping either hip.
- Inhale as you return the leg to the floor, and exhale as you lift the other leg.
- Do 10 repetitions.
- Inhale as you lower the leg, and exhale as you lower your hips back to the floor.

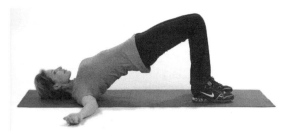

FIGURE 5.17

The Basic Bridge with Leg Extension

- Lie on your back with your knees bent and feet hip-distance apart.
- Focus on keeping your hips lifted and level.
- Inhale as you begin, and exhale as you lift your hips into a bridge position.
- Inhale as you hold this position, and exhale as you extend one leg toward the ceiling.
- Lower the leg so that it is parallel with the supporting leg, then lift the leg back to the ceiling and return it to the floor.
- Inhale as you return the leg to the floor, and exhale as you lift the other leg.
- Do 10 repetitions.

- Inhale as you lower the leg, and exhale as you lower your hips back to the floor. Start with the basic bridge first, and then progress to the full leg extension as your buttocks get stronger.

Taps

This exercise targets the gluteal muscles and strengthens the hips. It is great for golfers who tend to sway or slide.

- Lie on the floor on your left side. Form a straight line with your left leg, hip, and shoulder (see figure 5.18a).
- Bend the left elbow and place the left forearm on the floor.
- Bend the right knee and point the right foot so that your toes are pointing downward.
- Tap your toes on the floor directly behind the left knee.
- Rotate the right hip and tap your right knee on the floor directly in front of the knee (see figure 5.18b).
- Do 20 repetitions and switch sides.

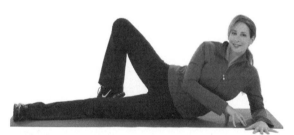

FIGURE 5.18A

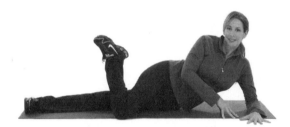

FIGURE 5.18B

■ Seniors Tee
FLEXIBILITY EQUALS LONGEVITY

As golfers play deeper into the "back nine of life," they tend to notice that in addition to losing bone density, muscle mass, memory, flexibility, and so forth, they discover that their drives start getting shorter, and their handicaps start getting higher. Desperate to remedy the situation, they will often go out and get that new state of the art driver or take a lesson from the local golf instructor who can teach them the latest "Tour move" that will get that extra distance back once and for all.

Despite the remarkable improvements in golf technology, golf instruction, and golf course conditioning, the truth is that all of this technology isn't going to grow the person with the AARP card a new hamstring or hip flexor. The most effective way to restore a senior's

STRETCHING DURING THE ROUND

We all know the importance of daily stretching, but do you know that you should also take the time to stretch during the round? Stretching while you play can help prevent your muscles from tightening up during the round, keep your muscles loose and supple, restore your spine angle, prevent injury, and help you swing more freely.

golf game is by instilling an effective flexibility program. No matter what the age, everyone can increase the range of motion in their bodies, if they stretch the right muscles the right way.

What is the proper stretching protocol for seniors? Stretching should always start with proper breathing. When a person breathes properly, oxygen will get deep into the nerve spindles and nerve fibers of the fascia, and as the fascia begins to relax, the muscle will begin to contract and expand more, hence it will gain more flexibility. A person who doesn't breathe properly and forces their stretch will actually prevent the oxygen from reaching the nerve spindles and create a myotatic stretch reflex, which will actually tighten the muscle.

The next step in proper stretching is recognizing the appropriate "muscle chains." Muscles run in chains, much like the shingles on a roof. Although they're all separate, they all interlock and flow together. For example, if one wants to stretch out a tight upper back, the place to start is usually with the calves, then the hamstrings, then the hips, the erectors, and finally the upper back and shoulders. Going straight to the shoulder is usually a waste of time, just like changing a flat tire that is really only flat due to the chassis being out of alignment. Without addressing the alignment problem in the chassis, the tire will only get flat again. Only when the chassis is properly aligned will the wheel turn over properly.

The third and final step in proper stretching is consistency. To counter the damaging effects of our sedentary life style, we must get into the habit of stretching on a daily basis. The good news is the more flexible you become, the less stretching you have to do.

JUNIOR GOLFERS AND RESISTANCE TRAINING

With all the buzz about golf fitness, you may be anxious to get your young golfer started with strength training to give him or her an edge over the competition; however, because their young bodies are still growing and developing, it is important to know what type of training your young athlete should be doing for his or her body type and age to keep them safe and injury free. "When it comes to conditioning for a prepubescent golfer, the best way to start them off is with light resistance loads using a variety of equipment, including elastic bands that come in progressive tensions, medicine balls, and even using their own body weight," says our own GFM advisory team member Dave Herman.

Herman, who trains the 2008 Masters champion Trevor Immelman and LPGA Tour sensation Suzann Pettersen, also coaches many young rising golf stars. He is currently training 14-year-old teen golf sensation Cindy Feng, who, since 2007, has won more than 10 tournaments on the Florida Junior Golf Tour and broke an AJGA record in 2008 for most consecutive wins in a single season. When Herman first started working with Feng, he had her doing lots of core stabilization and speed development exercises with elastic bands and elastic cords, having her focus on proper technique and form to learn at an early age how important technique is in protecting her body. When she turned 13, they transitioned into lifting dumbbells and cables to help her gain more strength while she continued working on and improving her game with her coach David Leadbetter. "Cindy is naturally flexible with a strong set of lower body wheels, so we are focusing on improving her rotational speed and upper body strength," says Herman.

When a junior golfer begins resistance training, it is important to choose activities that match their structural changes, genetics, and body type. According to Herman, "People assume that children are naturally flexible, but some kids may be tight because they don't stretch, because they have postural issues, or because of family genetics. We frequently begin their programs with neutral spine stabilization exercises and lots of band stretching to get the pelvis stable and exercises to improve joint flexibility to increase range of motion. Some kids may be naturally strong but need to work on decreasing body fat, so it is important to look at each child individually and design a program based on their needs."

Herman says that it is typically a good idea for younger children to stay away from heavier, high-risk weight training and begin strength training with light weights using push-pull exercises to create muscular tone and balance through the same planes. An example of a push-pull exercise is a dumbbell chest press followed by a dumbbell lat row. As the teenager grows older with a more solid athletic foundation, he or she can begin to move into higher-volume sets and advanced strength training exercises.

The following are a few rules that you should be aware of when it comes to exercise for children under the age of 18:

1. Consult your child's doctor before starting any exercise program.

2. Young golfers who are beginning to work out should get a proper assessment from a golf fitness trainer who has experience working with adolescents.

3. Children should begin by performing simple and basic low-risk exercises, concentrating on proper technique and form.

4. Children should exercise in an encouraging setting.

5. Children under the age of 13 should not lift heavy weights and should primarily use bands, medicine balls, and their own body weight to increase strength.

6. Children should always be properly supervised when exercising and lifting weights.

SUMMARY

The goal of this chapter is to present examples of golf-specific exercises that can help you get into golf shape and make you aware of the importance of fitness in golf. There is no one exercise or routine that will meet all your fitness needs. It is important to do a variety of exercises that incorporate building strength, flexibility, stability, and endurance specific to golf. The best way to start a golf fitness exercise program is to consult a golf fitness professional or golf teacher certified in golf fitness who can evaluate your fitness level and design a program to fit your needs.

10 TIPS FOR KEEPING YOU ON TRACK WITH YOUR GOLF-SPECIFIC WORKOUT

1. *Maintain consistency*. It is better to do a few minutes of golf-specific stretches each day than wait until you have a couple of hours free at the end of the week. It usually never happens.

2. *Work out in the morning before you play your round of golf*. You may be too tired afterward. Working out prior to your round will help you loosen your muscles.

3. *Set goals you can reach*. For example, decide to warm up before every round and practice session.

4. *Find a workout partner*. Get one of your golfing buddies to start a golf-specific fitness program with you.

5. *Walk while you play golf*. Walking rather than riding in a cart allows you to kill two birds with one stone: You can improve your fitness while you play.

6. *Find a fitness routine that you like and is easy to work into your busy schedule*. Keep some light weights, resistance bands, and an exercise ball in your bedroom so you can do a few exercises in the morning and before you go to bed.

7. *Combine strength training and aerobic exercise*. Instead of doing two separate workouts, combine weight training with cardiovascular exercises. It will speed up your workout.

8. *Hire a golf-specific fitness trainer*. This is especially important if you are just beginning your fitness program. GFM will soon unveil the International Golf Fitness Directory listing all the top fitness specialists in the world.

9. *Watch a sports movie*. The movie *The Greatest Game Ever Played* about 19-year-old Francis Quimet beating Harry Vardon, one of the greatest golfers ever to win the US Open, is a great motivational flick.

10. *Read GFM*. You will find the latest information on fitness, nutrition, and mental techniques from some of the best fitness experts and golf instructors in the world.

CHAPTER 6

WORK OUT LIKE THE PROS

Training with Trevor Immelman, Phil Mickelson, Justin Rose, and Suzann Pettersen

It is a well-known fact that in such sports as football, basketball, and tennis, professional athletes perform sport-specific training drills and exercises to prepare them for competition. In the last 10 years, professional golfers have come to realize the benefits of sport-specific training for golf and are now preparing themselves for their seasons much like other athletes do. And why wouldn't they? Professional golfers are athletes, too.

Although unseen to the general public, professional golfers spend countless hours off the golf course, in the gym, conditioning their bodies to perform at the highest level of competition by doing strength and endurance training and stretching. Before a tournament round, although behind the scenes, professional golfers take time to perform warm-up routines that include cardiovascular and limbering-up exercises to warm up muscles and joints, followed by golf-specific stretches and other drills to get the body ready to swing the club. This session happens even before they step onto the practice range. After the round, they may follow up with a postround flexibility program that stretches muscles and helps the body to recover from the twisting, squatting, and walking they did during the round. They also follow golf-specific training programs on their days off and during the off-season.

Fitness has become a staple in the professional golf world. The PGA, Senior PGA, and LPGA tours travel with fitness trailers equipped with licensed therapists, professional fitness trainers, and state-of-the-art machines for players to use during tournaments. The fitness trailer on the PGA Tour is a 44-foot semi with 2 sides that fold out. When fully extended, it covers more than 1,500 square feet. On any given day, dozens of tour players can be found on the various machines warming up, stretching, or performing their golf-specific workouts.

Professionals know the importance of maintaining themselves as finely tuned athletes to not only help them increase strength for power and distance, but also prevent injury and extend their playing careers. In this chapter, you will learn what PGA and LPGA tour professionals like Masters champion Trevor Immelman, six-time major winner Nick Faldo, and LPGA major winner Suzanne Pettersen are doing to achieve a stronger, more flexible body for a more powerful, smoother swing that can withstand the pressure of tournament golf week in and week out. Our GFM contributors also show you the routines they use with their professional clients to keep them in top golf shape. Whether you have been playing golf for years or you're just a beginner, improving your golf fitness is a must if you want to take your game to a higher level.

WORKING OUT WITH TREVOR IMMELMAN

During his off-season, GFM met up with 2008 Masters champion Trevor Immelman and his golf performance coach, Dave Herman, also a GFM contributor, who has been working with Immelman on his fitness since before his historic win. Immelman is a confident, athletic golfer who has followed the path of his boyhood idol and lifelong mentor Gary Player. Player has dedicated himself to continuously improving his physical and mental golf fitness, as well as the longevity of his career.

In winning his first major, Immelman, a native of South Africa with 10 worldwide wins, says that his confidence has reached a new level. "I definitely feel more confident. I have proved to myself that if I play my best, I can beat the best. I now fully believe that I can win the biggest tournaments."

After two physical setbacks in 2007—a stomach virus resulting in significant weight loss, and major surgery in December, only five months before his major win—Immelman's dedicated approach to fitness enabled him to get in form and win the Masters. "I found how important it is to have a trainer as good as Dave Herman who knows how to prepare an athlete in terms of strength and nutrition," said Immelman. Immelman has tweaked his routine during the tournament season by using lighter weights, simple core stabilization, and more elastic stretching. The focus is on staying pain free, loose, and limber for tournament play and not lifting heavier weights, which could cause too much stiffness.

Immelman, who turned pro at age 20, feels that overall fitness is crucial in extending his career in professional golf. He says, "Golf is such a different animal than other sports when it comes to training. With other sports, like football or baseball, you are lucky to have a 10-year window, so you have got to hit it with your maximum training. In the sport of golf, your training is more centered on preventing injuries and adding longevity to your game and your career. It is a sport where you want to play competitively until you are 50 or 60. You just need to be fit enough to play 72 holes, never lose concentration, never get tired, and enable your body and muscles to support your swing, all in an effort to avoid injury. It's a little different balance than any other sport, and that's how Dave and I got onto this angle for golf-specific conditioning and the workout we are going to show you today."

And what does Gary Player have to say about all of this? If you recall, Player had some inspirational words for Immelman the night before his final round at the 2008 Masters, and he regularly stays in touch with Immelman. During their last conversation, Player explained how he was working on some new conditioning techniques that he felt he needed to add to his regimen for his aging and changing body. Immelman finds it fascinating and inspiring that at age 75, Player still looks for ways to improve. "It just shows what a positive attitude he has. We are always talking about golf fitness and discussing conditioning techniques and stuff. He always gives me a slap in the abs just to see how I am doing," said Immelman.

Immelman, who is actually a great study of golf-specific fitness himself, used the aid of Herman to assemble an awesome workout routine that practically anyone can safely do on their own. Herman has worked with Immelman, one of the Tour's most fitness-dedicated athletes, for quite some time perfecting golf-specific exercises. These exercises encompass all of the important aspects of the golf swing for more strength, speed, and, most importantly, longevity.

Knowing that training for golf is different from any other sport, Immelman and Herman formulated a routine that promotes being completely balanced during the swing. Immelman assured us that "when you play a downhill lie, you will notice a difference in your stability." They designed a core stabilization program consistent with building and maintaining leg, upper body, and core strength, all aspects that promote an automatically balanced swing, as well as a reduced risk of injury. This is a whole upper body and leg program that is performed while keeping the core muscles engaged and firing throughout the entire workout.

The routine we outline for you is an abbreviated version of a more intensive workout that lasts up to 90 minutes for Immelman. Based on time limitations to balance his professional and personal life, he divides it into two 45-minute sessions. For the purposes of the routine designed for you, 30 minutes is all that is necessary to get through the exercises. Herman suggests a 10-minute cool down walk and light stretching to keep your muscles loose and long. Plan on maximizing the weights to a degree where you can still continue to focus on keeping your core engaged. This makes the routine safe for any healthy golfer. "This program is all about minimizing the risk of injury to your back, both in the gym and on the course," explains Herman.

Begin by using lighter weights. Work your way up to heavier weights as you strengthen your core muscles. Although it may appear that there isn't much to the routine, the moves involved will markedly strengthen the hundreds of tiny muscles that stabilize the center of your body, not to mention your upper body and legs. If you have not already participated in a program that conditions your core muscles, be sure to step into this lightly. Expect some instability and wobble with your body in the beginning. As you improve your strength, you will notice that your stabilization skills will improve automatically for better body control. This stabilization process is the result of strengthened muscles that are needed to create a more balanced and safe swing, which, of course, means more distance, lower scores, and added longevity to your game.

The Core and Core Stabilization

The main muscles involved in core stabilization are deep muscles, including the transverse abdominus muscles, multifidus muscles, and muscles of the pelvic floor. When engaged, the transverse abdominus creates a protective barrier around your spine. It's the deep lower abdominal muscle you work if you pull in your belly button toward your stomach while exhaling the air in the diaphragm. The multifidus is a muscle that lies along your spine from your neck to your pelvis, with short fibers connecting one bone (vertebra) of the spine to other vertebrae near it. The muscles of the pelvic floor are most noticeable when you squeeze to keep yourself from urinating.

These muscles, along with muscles closer to the surface, help with core stabilization and posture, and they also help you move more efficiently. The muscles closer to the surface include the thoracic area of the upper back, musculature of the lower back, and multiple gluteus muscles. Musculature connected to the pelvic muscles that also help stabilize the body include quads/lateral I-t bands, adductors, and hip flexors. Core stabilization strengthens the body and helps you learn to use the inner muscles that create a strong, protective, and balanced center linking the upper and lower body, which is optimum for golf.

Immelman's Core Stabilization Workout

Equipment you will need for this workout includes the following:

- ankle bands
- looped resistance band
- stability ball
- dumbbells
- yoga brick
- Bosu ball
- medicine ball
- Pilates ring (optional)

As you begin this workout, it is important to understand exactly what core stabilization is and the importance of keeping your center (core) engaged like a vacuum around your spine to maintain the pelvis in a neutral and safe position throughout each exercise. If you are not regularly doing this type of training program or are suffering from a lower back injury, consult your physician, physical therapist, or personal trainer before starting this exercise routine.

THE WARM-UP

Do a 10- to 20-minute warm-up using a treadmill, stationary bike, or elliptical machine. Follow with a light stretching routine or dynamic stretching routine with a looped resistance band, if possible.

1. THE ABDOMINAL STABILIZATION EXERCISE ON A STABILITY BALL

- Attach one end of a resistance band to a stable object behind you or have someone hold it for you.
- Sit on top of a stability ball.

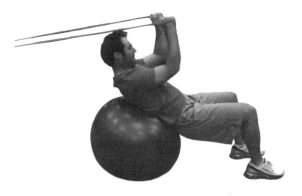

FIGURE 6.1

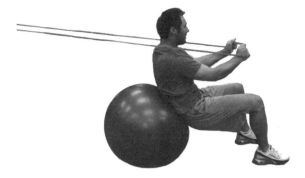

FIGURE 6.2

- Perform abdominal crunches, focusing on rolling from a horizontal to a vertical position (see figure 6.1).
- Hold at the top of the move (see figure 6.2).
- Follow this holding movement with a set of short, rapid repetitions, exhaling with each repetition.
- Do 2 sets, holding for 15 seconds at the top of each move.
- Do 1 set of 10 full-range crunches at a quick pace.

2. THE CHEST-ALTERNATING DUMBBELL EXERCISE ON A STABILITY BALL

- Place an ankle band around the lower legs to engage the lateral muscles of the upper legs, while also engaging the gluteal muscles (buttocks) and abdominal muscles.
- Lie on a stability ball with your shoulder blades centered on the ball (see figure 6.3).
- Focus on engaging your abdominal muscles to maintain a bridge position.
- Alternate single-arm chest presses using your dumbbells (see figures 6.4 and 6.5). Start out with light weights until you get stronger to

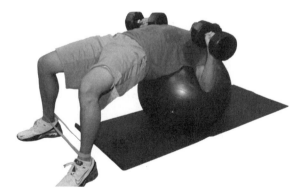

FIGURE 6.3

maintain proper technique and keep your core muscles engaged throughout the exercise.

- Extend and retract each arm fully before changing arms. You should feel the center of your body shifting slightly from side to side while performing the move.
- Do 2 sets of 30 repetitions (15 repetitions with each arm).

3. THE STANDING SINGLE-LEG SHOULDER PRESS

It is important to keep the core engaged throughout this entire exercise. As you engage the center of your body, keep the spine straight and the pelvis in a neutral position before lifting the weight above your head.

- Place an ankle band around the lower legs to engage the lateral muscles of the upper legs and hips.
- Stand with one leg on the floor (or on a yoga brick for added difficulty), and keep the supporting leg slightly bent (see figure 6.6).
- Begin with the dumbbell elevated in shoulder press position (see figure 6.7).
- Press the dumbbell up and down in a slow, steady motion while maintaining a strong stable core and balancing on one leg (see figure 6.8).

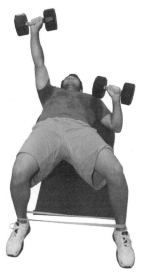

FIGURE 6.4

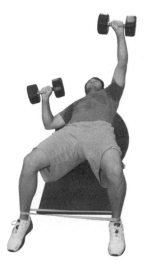

FIGURE 6.5

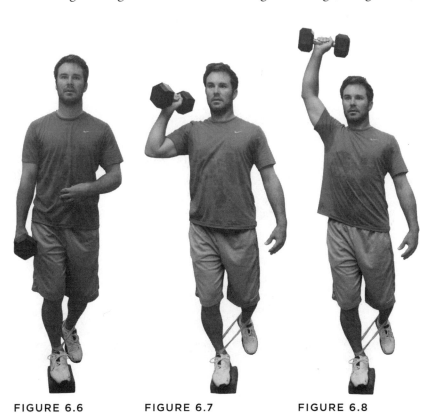

FIGURE 6.6   FIGURE 6.7   FIGURE 6.8

Use a light to medium weight so that you can focus on core stabilization throughout the exercise.

- Do 2 sets of 12 repetitions on each leg.

4. THE PLANK EXERCISE WITH ENHANCED STABILIZATION

This exercise can be performed with varying levels of difficulty (as pictured) for more intensity. Immelman describes it as a "killer of an exercise for the golfer."

- Start with your elbows and feet directly on the floor.
- Lift the rest of your body up off of the floor.
- Pull your abdominal muscles toward the spine, while keeping your pelvis and gluteal muscles aligned with the rest of your body. This is known as the plank position. Make your best effort to hold the plank position, and be careful not to let your neck drop down too much.
- Focus on an object in front of you, remembering to inhale and exhale as you hold the position.
- Repeat this move twice for a duration of 20 seconds each, gradually building up to holding for one minute.
- Use the Bosu ball for even more difficulty (see figure 6.9). Place a yoga brick underneath your toes to add additional instability opposing the Bosu ball (see figure 6.10). Add a medicine ball underneath your feet for the highest level of difficulty (see figures

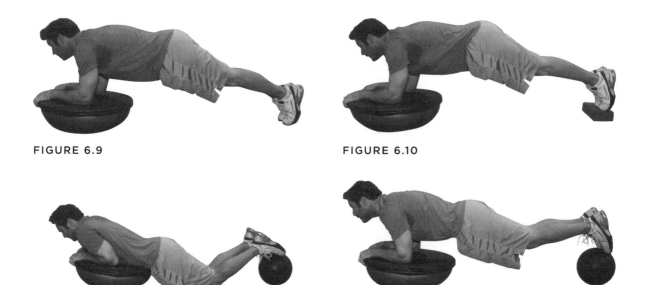

FIGURE 6.9

FIGURE 6.10

FIGURE 6.11

FIGURE 6.12

6.11 and 6.12). Work toward the more advanced levels to enhance the firing of your core stabilization muscles.

5. THE CORE BRIDGE ON A STABILITY BALL WITH LEG EXTENSION

- Lie on a stability ball with your shoulder blades centered on the ball.
- Focus on engaging your abdominal muscles to maintain a bridge position, exhaling as you hold a stable and centered position.
- Slowly extend your right leg so that it forms a straight line with the rest of your body (see figure 6.13).
- Hold for a three-second count while taking small, short breaths.
- Release the leg slowly to the floor.
- Restabilize the core and repeat the move with the other leg.
- Use caution, as this exercise is more difficult than it appears. It may take a few workouts to get your body under control. Start with three repetitions on each leg, and hold the leg extension for three seconds. Build to five repetitions on each leg, holding each leg extended for a five-second count.

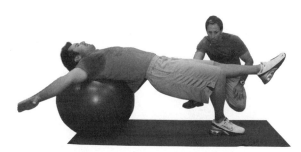

FIGURE 6.13

6. THE DUAL/SINGLE-LEG HAMSTRING CURL

- Lie with your back flat on the floor.
- Move into a bridge position, with your legs straight and your heels on top of the stability ball (see figure 6.14).
- Roll the ball toward your buttocks until your feet are flush against the ball (see figure 6.15).
- Slowly return to the starting position.
- To make the move more difficult, hold a weight disk or medicine ball in your hands (see figure 6.16). For added intensity, use only one leg at a time, while slightly elevating the other leg up off of the ball (see figure 6.17). For even more intensity, use only one leg at a time and hold the opposite leg in a vertical position (see figure 6.18).

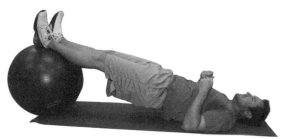

FIGURE 6.14

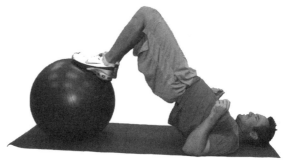

FIGURE 6.15

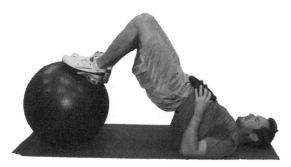

FIGURE 6.16

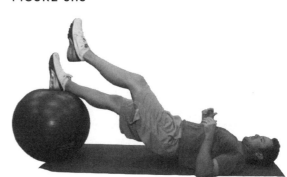

FIGURE 6.17

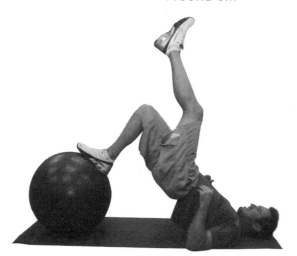

FIGURE 6.18

- Repeat the move with the opposite leg.
- Start with 8 repetitions and build to 15.

7. CORE ROTATION WITH STABILIZATION

This exercise is a basic core rotation movement that Herman has modified to increase core stability and recruit the fast twitch muscle fibers, the fibers of the muscle that contract quickly and powerfully, in the abdominal and oblique muscles. The move can be performed simply by using the looped resistance band for a good rotation exercise; however, you can greatly intensify the effectiveness for all of the core muscles by adding the ankle band and Pilates ring.

- Place the resistance band around a stable object and stand sideways.
- Grab the free end of the band with both hands.
- Rotate the shoulders and chest until they are centered with your hips.
- Hold for 15 seconds.
- Repeat 1 or 2 times on each side, holding each time for 15 seconds.
- Add the ankle band to engage the lower body (see figure 6.19). Add the Pilates ring to engage more of the upper body (see figure 6.20).

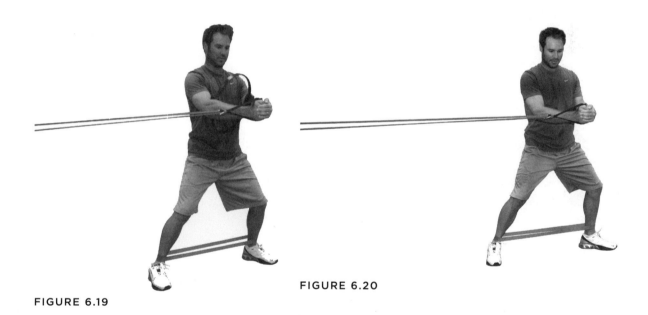

FIGURE 6.20

FIGURE 6.19

Speed and Flexibility

Another aspect of golf fitness that Immelman wanted to address was speed and flexibility. A few years ago, Herman started Immelman on a training program he calls Athleticity™ that combines elasticity, flexibility, and core strength training. The program uses specialized flex band training that has become a revolutionary new performance tool for golfers of all ages and abilities. These flex bands are called Super-Flex™ bands.

While initially designed for athletes, these bands are extremely effective for people of all ages. Anyone who wants to stay flexible, increase strength, and reduce the incidence of "aches and pains" as they get older will benefit from band training. SuperFlex™ bands are also great for adolescents because they are fun, safe, and create less compression on growth plates and joints. SuperFlex™ band training is an inexpensive and highly effective way of achieving a more physically fit body. It is well documented that resistance training can improve muscular strength and local muscular endurance, increase flexibility and power, and stimulate positive effects on the body.

Using this concept of Athleticity™, Herman developed a golf-specific program with Immelman's help. The team wanted to change the focus from building muscle and adding weight to introducing more speed and flexibility. As the result of applying Athleticity™ to Immelman's program, they were able to increase his athleticism, strength, and elasticity. Immelman believes that the bands have increased his speed, flexibility, and power, and he has no doubt that the bands have helped take his fitness to the next level.

Immelman's Speed and Flexibility Workout

THE WARM-UP

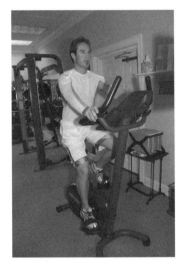

FIGURE 6.21

Start with a 5- to 10-minute preworkout warm-up. A 5- to 10-minute ride on a stationary bike (see figure 6.21) or a brisk walk prior to working out is essential to warming up your muscles to help decrease the risk of injury and stiffness. Increase your ride to 45 minutes for a more cardiovascular workout.

THE SHOULDER STRETCH

This is an excellent golf-specific stretch for the upper back and shoulders. It mimics the shoulder turn at the top of the backswing. Good shoulder rotation helps take the stress off of your lower back, especially with the follow-through. As you lean into the stretch, the band lengthens, allowing you to control the tension, resulting in a deeper and longer stretch throughout the targeted area.

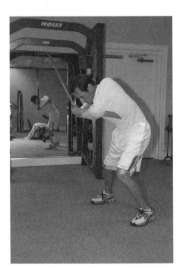

FIGURE 6.22

- Loop one end of a medium-width band around a bar or other stable object and the other end of the band around your left wrist.
- Bend the left knee (the knee farthest from the band) and lean into the stretch. Focus on releasing and lengthening the left shoulder and upper back (deltoid and lat) muscles (see figure 6.22).
- Repeat the stretch on the opposite side.

THE FRONTAL PLANE STRETCH

This stretch targets the hip flexor, abdominal, and chest muscles. It is a great stretch along the frontal plane of the body, which tends to be shortened and tight in most active golfers. The use of bands helps control the tension of the stretch. Looser hip flexors will help promote a better hip turn, and more flexibility in the chest area will allow you to assume a better position at the top of the backswing. Flexibility in both of these positions will help take the stress off of the lower back.

- Attach one end of a flex band to the right ankle and the other end to a stable object.
- Attach one end of another flex band to the left wrist and the other end to a stable object.
- Press the weight of the rest of your body forward, placing your right hand on the floor for support (see figure 6.23).
- Repeat the stretch on the opposite side.

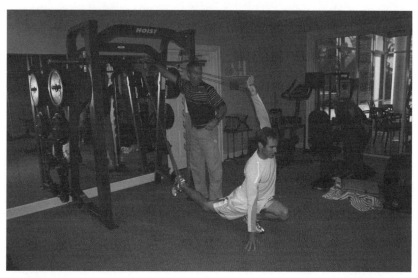

FIGURE 6.23

THE OVERHEAD TRICEPS EXTENSION

In figures 6.24 and 6.25, Immelman is performing an advanced triceps extension using a cable and an ultralight band. While doing this exercise, the addition of a flex band dynamically increases the tension, allowing you to accelerate and fire through the movement to develop strength and speed in the muscles. This will add power to your downswing.

- Loop the flex band around the cable handle and apparatus bar or any stable object.

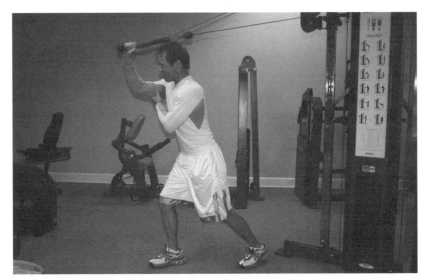

FIGURE 6.24

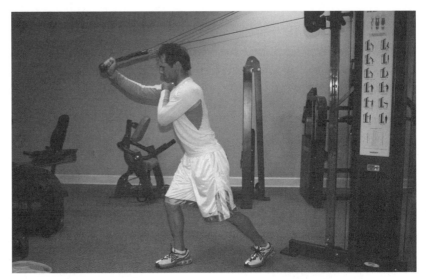

FIGURE 6.25

- Begin with your elbow bent at a 90-degree angle, and extend the arm forward. As you extend through the movement, the band tension increases, causing the stabilizer muscles in your shoulder and triceps to work even harder.
- Do 3 sets of 10 repetitions on each arm.

BICEP CURLS

This exercise works on symmetry and arm strength. Having balanced muscles in the arm, including your triceps and biceps, is key in maintaining an overall athletic body. Good symmetrical arm strength is also a great preventative measure against the stresses that can cause irritation and injury to the elbow. The use of flex bands is important in this exercise because of their ability to maintain tension at the end of the movement. As the flex band pulls at the end of this movement, it helps keep the biceps stretched and flexible. Strong biceps, and even biceps with some bulk, are okay for the golfer, as long as they stay flexible.

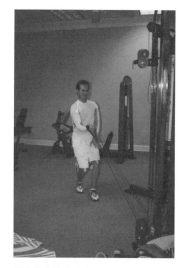

FIGURE 6.26

- Loop the flex band around a stable object.
- Grasp the band with the palm of your hand facing upward (see figure 6.26).
- Contract your arm toward your chest, stopping at 45 degrees rather than bringing your arm the whole way up to your chest.
- Release and fully extend the arm.
- Do 3 sets of 10 repetitions on each arm.

SHOULDER TS

This is an excellent preventative exercise that strengthens the small muscles that protect the rotator cuff. It also develops upper body strength in the rear deltoids that helps develop good golf posture. Strong shoulders will add power to the golf swing and help hold the right position at the top of the backswing. Since there is an immense amount of force created during the downswing and impact, having strong shoulders is a great way to prevent golf-specific injuries.

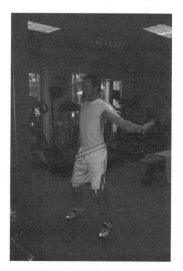

FIGURE 6.27

- Attach one end of an ultralight band around each wrist and the other end to a stationary bar or other object.
- Maintain the wrists at the level of the thighs.
- Draw each wrist to the shoulders.
- Place another band around the ankles to improve core stabilization by engaging the leg, hip, and deep core muscles (see figure 6.27).
- Do 3 sets of 10 repetitions.

THE MILITARY PRESS

This is one of the heavier exercises that can be done to develop more strength and muscle mass and promote an overall balanced athletic body. The use of the flex bands is important because it makes the exercise more fluid and difficult.

- Sit down at a shoulder press machine with your feet shoulder-width apart.

- Wrap one end of a flex band around the top of the bar of the machine and the other end around the bottom, or have someone step on the band to hold it in place (see figure 6.28).
- Press the bar up as you exhale. Extend your arms fully at the top of the move.
- Pull the bar down to the starting position. The change in the tension at the top of the movement pulls the weight down faster than gravity alone. This promotes speed in the downward movement and helps recruit the eccentric fast twitch fibers in the muscle.
- Do 3 sets of 10 repetitions and switch arms.

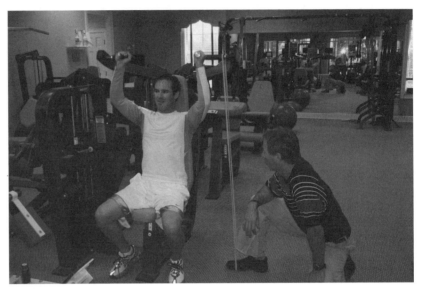

FIGURE 6.28

THE HIGH CABLE PULL

This exercise strengthens the posterior shoulder muscles and works the core muscles through the same plane as the golf swing. Proper movement and strength in these muscles is crucial for power and stability in the movement. In addition to the cable, flex bands are attached to add resistance to the exercise. Because we use a natural movement, it is a good, safe exercise for the rear deltoids and increasing core strength.

- Wrap a flex band around the top of a cable rack.
- Grasp the band with your right hand with your palm facing downward.
- Bend the left knee and extend the left leg forward to maintain your balance.

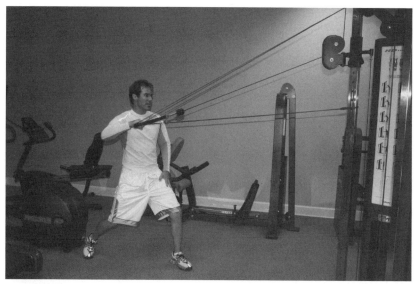

FIGURE 6.29

- Extend the right arm and pull the band toward you so that your right elbow is aligned with your right side (see figure 6.29).
- Return to the starting position.
- Do 3 sets of 10 repetitions and switch arms.

ABDOMINAL CRUNCHES

Using a band during an abdominal crunch while sitting on a stability ball increases development of upper and lower abdominal as well as oblique muscles. Using a band allows you to control the tension for a more dynamic core strengthening exercise. Core strength is a key element in protecting the spine, creating speed, and stabilizing the body.

- Wrap one end of a stability band around a stationary object.
- Lie on your back on a stability ball with your knees bent and holding the free end of the band above your head with your elbows bent.
- Contract your abdominal muscles as you lift toward the ceiling (see figure 6.30).
- Do 3 sets of 10 repetitions.

WORKING OUT WITH PHIL MICKELSON

After shedding a few unwanted pounds, Phil Mickelson went on to shed the title of the "best golfer in the world not to have won a major"

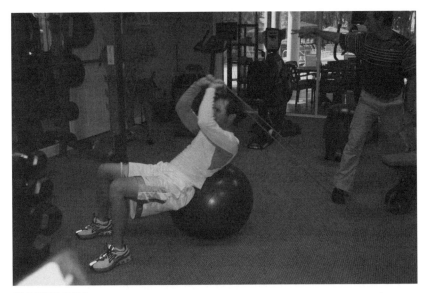

FIGURE 6.30

when he captured the 2004 Masters. But after a few years, Mickelson, who readily admits to indulging in fried food and letting his fitness regimen slide, recommitted himself to fitness and a healthier diet, resulting in a lighter, healthier, happier Phil with the start of the 2007 golf season. "At the end of the 2006 season, I know he was quoted as saying that he got away from his golf fitness training to a degree during the year, and that may have affected his play as the year progressed," says Sean Cochran, Mickelson's fitness trainer. The world's number 2 player returned to action 20 pounds lighter with the help of Cochran, who devised a specific program for Mickelson to help him increase flexibility, balance, strength, and power for more clubhead speed and to combat fatigue. "Once the younger players started to come on tour, Phil realized that he had to start working out to maintain longevity in his career," Cochran explains.

Mickelson's fitness regime is based on a "periodization" system in which Cochran divides the year into three different training stages. "We have an off-season program where the intensity and volume of his training is high, a preseason program where the volume and intensity is moderate, and an in-season program where the volume is low and intensity moderate," explains Cochran. During the preseason portion of the program, Cochran lowers the training intensity to allow Mickelson more time to practice and work on his game to prepare for tournaments. During the competitive season, the program moves to in-season training mode, where the volume of exercise is less than his off-season and the training intensity is moderate. "This allows Phil to maintain the physical gains developed during the off-season, as well as be prepared to play competitively week in and week out," says Cochran.

Mickelson's commitment to fitness helps him increase flexibility for greater range of motion in the golf swing, strengthen the lower body and core to help maintain proper posture and swing positions, and increase power for more distance. Along with exercise, Mickelson changed his diet, which helped speed up his metabolism, resulting in weight loss. Mickelson now eats four to five small meals of protein and vegetables during the day, and he has cut out junk food. During the off-season, a typical week of training consists of 4 to 5 days of aerobic conditioning for 30 to 45 minutes and a 1-hour strength training session.

The following exercises are part of one of Mickelson's training routines designed by Cochran. Equipment you will need for this workout includes the following:

- Physioball

Rotators

- Place your feet shoulder-width apart, extend your arms overhead, clasp your hands together, and look straight ahead.
- Slowly extend your hands toward the tops of your feet.
- Extend downward until you can feel a stretch in your hamstrings and lower back (see figure 6.31).
- Pause for one second and return to the starting position.
- Rotate your torso, shoulders, arms, and head to the right.
- Extend your hands downward to the outside of the right foot.
- Pause for one second and return to the starting position.
- Repeat the same sequence to your left.
- Perform 10 to 15 repetitions.

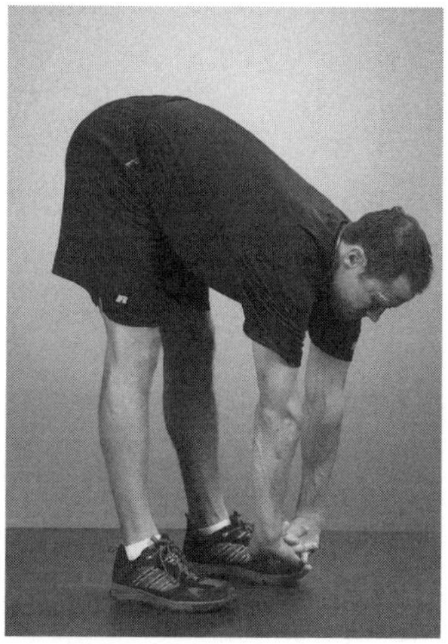

FIGURE 6.31

The Physioball Russian Twist

- Place your head and shoulders on top of the Physioball.
- Elevate the hips so that they align with your knees and shoulders.
- Place your feet on the floor shoulder-width apart, extend the arms straight out in front of your chest, and clasp your hands together.
- Rotate to the left, allowing the ball to roll underneath your shoulders. Allow the eyes to follow your hands during the rotation.

- Continue to rotate to the left until your left upper arm is resting on top of the ball.
- Return to the starting position.
- Repeat the rotation to your right.
- Alternate the rotation left and right for 15 to 20 repetitions.

The Single-Leg Airplane Rotation

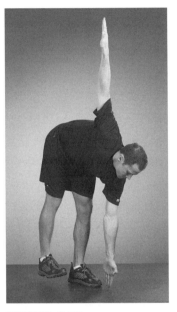

- Place your feet together and bend at the hips so that your back is flat and your chest is parallel with the floor.
- Extend your arms out to the side.
- Lift the right foot off of the floor, and balance on your left foot. Keep the right foot off the floor for the entire exercise.
- Rotate your left arm downward toward the left foot while simultaneously rotating the right arm upward toward the ceiling (see figure 6.32), creating the rotation in the torso of your body.
- Continue to rotate until the left hand is directly above your left foot and the right hand is pointing upward toward the ceiling.
- Return to the starting position.
- Do 10 to 15 repetitions and repeat the sequence balancing on your right foot.

FIGURE 6.32

WORKING OUT WITH JUSTIN ROSE

One look at PGA Tour player Justin Rose and you can tell that this top-ranked player knows the importance of golf fitness. You can also ascertain that it is not something he takes lightly. As a matter of fact, golf fitness is something that he knows has enabled him to keep playing the game that he loves and keep playing it well. At 28 years of age, Rose has been through more than some of the most senior PGA Tour players, both mentally and physically, and he has continued to impress the golf world with his charisma and charm on and off of the golf course.

Diagnosed with a bulging disk in his lower back more than six years ago, Rose was faced with the fact that the condition of his back could ultimately end his short-lived career. Around this time, he began working with expert sports injury trainer and physiotherapist Kam Bhabra. Bhabra, who is decorated with a list of degrees, certifications, and honors in the field of sports injury and physical therapy, saw to it that Rose got the best possible treatment for his bulging disk, as well as a plan to prevent further back injury.

Six years later, as a result of his treatment, Rose is at the top of his game, and his back is strong and fit. The type of golf-specific fitness that Rose has incorporated into his daily routine was based on Bhabra's program that, in the beginning, involved intense physical therapy to prevent surgery. Today his routine consists of total performance training to continue to strengthen the areas around his bulging disk and keep his back in posture-perfect shape.

Explaining Bhabra's Principles

The following three principles form the basis for Rose's daily workout routine:

1. *Maintain a perfect platform.* Your platform is how you set up your swing and maintain your stability while swinging the club. A proper platform will channel your power and give you control. A proper setup simply means starting your swing in the right place so you can finish in the right place. To have a proper setup, you need to have the correct posture to create a perfect platform. This will greatly reduce the chances of injuring or reinjuring your back.

2. *Remember the x-factor.* The x-factor is defined by how well you keep your hips straight and relaxed (or in a neutral position) in contrast to how you turn your shoulders and upper core during your swing. By keeping your hips straight and turning with your upper body, you are alleviating any stress or strain on your lower back caused by the power in your swing.

3. *Build a strong core.* A true core workout is one that focuses on the abdominal region; however, it should also develop key muscles attached to your hips, pelvic region, and lower back. A strong, solid core results in proper form or posture and reduces your chance of injury. Without proper posture, injury can occur. In Rose's case, he suffers from an excessive anterior pelvic tilt, or protruding backside. This is commonly referred to as S-posture. Maintaining a strong core is crucial for Rose to prevent his bulging disk from flaring up.

Now that we have the theory behind Rose's golf-specific workout, let's take a look at some of the drills that Bhabra does with Rose to enable him to manage his injury. These simple moves are something that any golfer can do at home, in the gym, or traveling, and they are primarily used to strengthen the core muscles in the abdominal region. The following is just one of the workout routines that Rose does on a weekly basis, and this one focuses primarily on the core region. Wearing the TechFit PowerWeb undergarment by Adidas, Justin explained that this "posture guard," as he referred to it, is an excellent way to remind him to keep his posture perfect while swinging the club or working out.

Rose's Circuit Workout for the Core Region

Equipment you will need for this workout includes the following:

- exercise mat

THE WARM-UP AND DRILLS 1 AND 2

- Sit on your knees and stretch your hands out in front of you, reaching forward as far as you can (see figure 6.33). Feel the deep stretch all along the back.
- Return to a flat position on your mat with your face down and your hands positioned in front of you.
- Slowly begin to lift your head and feet up off of the mat without arching your back (see figure 6.34).
- Hold for 60 seconds and repeat the move. You should be able to increase the time that you hold this position on a weekly basis. In Rose's case, he has built up to 20 repetitions. Start out by doing 2 to 3 repetitions, and work toward increasing to 20.

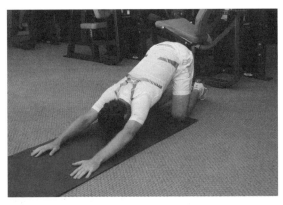

FIGURE 6.33

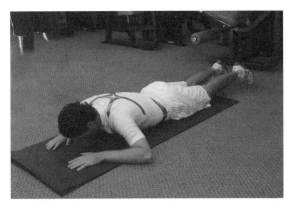

FIGURE 6.34

DRILL 3

- Lie on your back and bend at the knees while keeping your upper back pressed firmly against the mat.
- Slowly raise one leg up and point your toes toward the ceiling. Keep your hands on your stomach and the raised leg parallel with the bent knee (see figure 6.35).

- Hold the move for 60 seconds and repeat.
- Increase the length of time that you hold the position as you strengthen your core and the surrounding muscles. Do not strain while performing the move, as it could lead to injury.

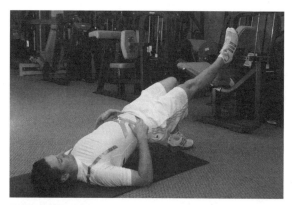

FIGURE 6.35

DRILL 4

Rose refers to this move as the "Ab Burn."

- Lie on the mat face down in a neutral position.
- Lift your body up off of the mat.
- Squeeze your abdominal muscles and keep your buttocks and back evenly aligned. Squeeze your shoulder blades together.
- Hold the position for 30 seconds (see figure 6.36). (Justin has it mastered at 2 minutes.) Do not allow your lower back to arch (see Bhabra next to Rose in figure 6.37 demonstrating the wrong way to do this drill). Bhabra is allowing his back to arch in the middle,

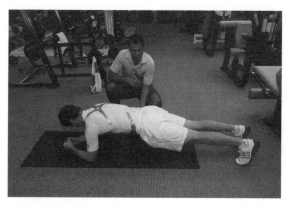

FIGURE 6.36

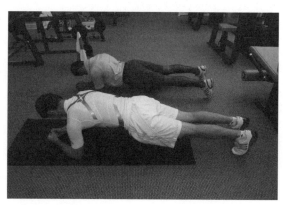

FIGURE 6.37

which causes extreme stress on the lower back. Rose is keeping his body level with his shoulders and has complete control of his back.

DRILL 5

- Lie on your stomach with your legs together and arms out to the side (see figure 6.38).
- Lift your head slightly up off of the mat.
- Raise your hands above your head and move your legs into a V position (see figure 6.39).
- Return to the starting position.
- Repeat this move for 30 seconds.
- Repeat one to two times, increasing the number of repetitions each week.

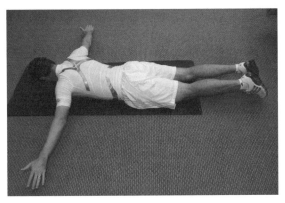

FIGURE 6.38

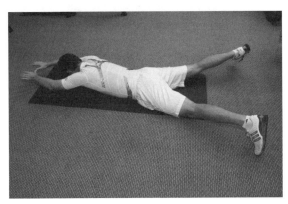

FIGURE 6.39

DRILL 6

Coordination is the key to this last drill. This exercise is about building your core to reduce injury.

- Lie face down on the mat.
- Gently lift your head and left arm up off of the mat. Your left arm should be extended straight out in front of you.
- Raise your right leg (see figure 6.40). Be sure to keep your lower abdomen pressed firmly on the mat.
- Hold the move for 30 seconds.
- Repeat the move with the right arm extended straight out in front of you and the left leg elevated.
- Hold for 30 seconds.
- Do two to three sets with each leg to start, and work your way up to doing additional sets.

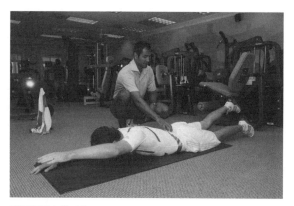

FIGURE 6.40

WORKING OUT WITH SUZANN PETTERSEN

Just as Tiger Woods works to perform his best in the majors, LPGA Tour player Suzann Pettersen has been working hard on her fitness and game to perform her best in the majors. The winner of five LPGA events, including a major at the McDonald's LPGA Championship, Pettersen has focused her attention on winning big tournaments. We at GFM have had the thrill of watching Pettersen improve her body, mind, and spirit over the last several years with a complete fitness makeover, one that concentrates on the mental as well as the physical side of her game, ultimately perfecting her performance, preventing injury, and creating longevity in her career.

When we first met Pettersen, she was with one of our GFM Advisory Team members, Lynn Teachworth, who is nationally and internationally recognized as one of the leaders in Structural Integration Neuromuscular Therapy. Teachworth's forte is in blending all styles of different muscle energy techniques, incorporating Body Talk, Reiki, acupuncture, and massage therapy in an effort to get the body and all of its systems working in perfect harmony. Pettersen has been working with Teachworth for more than three years and has found that the Structural Integration techniques Teachworth has used with her have enabled her to be in total control of her body.

Pettersen has long suffered from lower back problems, but after incorporating sports-specific massage and the holistic system of soft tissue manipulation, she feels that it has given her the opportunity to be in control of her pain, and not let the pain control her. So just what is structural integration, and how does it apply to total golf-specific fitness?

Formally referred to as Rolfing Structural Integration, the technique was discovered more than 50 years ago, when Dr. Ida P. Rolf realized that she could make remarkable changes in posture and structure by manipulating the body's myofascial system (the soft tissue or area located between the skin and the underlying structure of muscle and bone). It is a system of connective tissue that covers and connects the muscles, organs, and skeletal structures in the body. Muscle and fascia are united, forming the myofascial system.

This form of manipulation has the ability to dramatically alter a person's posture and structure. Athletes, especially golfers, have benefited tremendously from this pain and stress relief. In Pettersen's case, this treatment has created a more efficient use of the muscles her body needs to allow her to conserve energy, resulting in less fatigue on the course, while at the same time creating a more refined and relaxed movement in her swing.

"Working with Lynn and keeping massage and other holistic therapies in my routine, I feel that I have more awareness about my body and am more connected. I am in total control of my body, and this truly helps me on and off the course," explains Pettersen. She continues, saying, "I have always been extremely interested in the body, and if I were not a golfer, I would have been a physical therapist. So, to me, this type of therapy not only makes sense, it's natural."

Another benefit of golf-specific massage incorporated with Structural Integration is the way it increases the range of motion and improves total body balance, which is vital for any golfer. In Pettersen's case, Teachworth uses manual massage techniques that stretch out the fascia and restore tissues to optimum health, creating a synergy between muscle, tissue, and bone.

Pettersen also adds another vital component to her total performance routine: her daily workout with her fitness trainer, Dave Herman, who, as we already know, also trains 2008 Masters champion Trevor Immelman. Herman has transformed Pettersen's routine into one comprised of cardio (running/biking), daily resistance band workouts, stretching routines, medicine ball work, and core strengthening. Bands are an integral part of Pettersen's conditioning program, especially when she is on the road. Bands are lightweight, take up little space in luggage, and can be easily used in hotel rooms. Stretching and strengthening with bands creates more flexibility, less bulk, and less stress on joints and ligaments. Bands like the ones used by Pettersen can be purchased at sporting goods stores or online.

The following exercises can be used to warm up and wake up your muscles prior to a round of golf or simply maintain your physical condition while traveling on the road or at home before you play. Pettersen generally performs 1 to 2 sets of 8 to 10 repetitions for warming up and 2 to 3 sets of 12 to 20 repetitions for strengthening.

Equipment you will need for this workout includes the following:

- thin resistance band
- stability ball

The Total Shoulder

Pettersen uses a thin band to warm up and stretch her shoulders and upper back. This exercise can also be used to strengthen the shoulders and measure your range of motion while checking for any impingements or soreness that might have occurred the day before.

- Using a thin band, hold one end of the band in one hand and the other end in the opposite hand.
- Raise your arms above your head and stretch (see figure 6.41).
- Rotate your arms behind your back and stretch (see figure 6.42).
- Then move your arms in front of your chest and stretch (see figure 6.43).
- Return to the starting position.
- Repeat the sequence for 10 to 20 seconds.

Upper Body Stretching

Pettersen uses a thin band to stretch her chest, shoulder, and back muscles. Keeping these muscles elastic and free will help decrease the chance of injury and increase speed and stability.

- Wrap a band around a stable object at a level higher than your head, or have someone hold one end while you hold the other in your right hand (see figure 6.44).
- Stand up straight and extend the right arm over your head, leaning to the left side until you feel the stretch in your right chest, shoulder, and back muscles (see figure 6.45).
- Return to starting position.
- Perform 10 repetitions and switch sides.

The Rotational Core

Herman holds a thin resistance band while Pettersen performs a rotational core movement to warm up the muscles used in the golf swing. This is an excellent exercise to engage the core and loosen up the lower back.

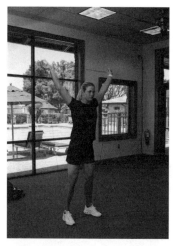

FIGURE 6.41

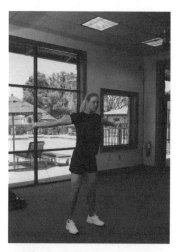

FIGURE 6.42

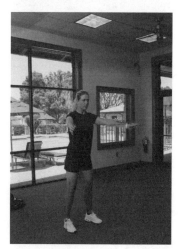

FIGURE 6.43

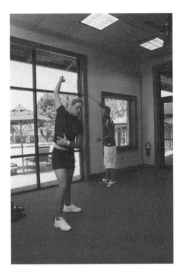

FIGURE 6.44

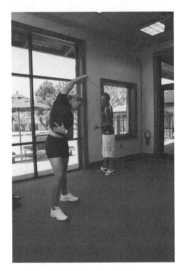

FIGURE 6.45

- Wrap one end of a resistance band around a stationary object or have someone hold the end for you.
- Stand sideways with the right arm facing the band and the left arm facing away from the band.
- Holding the free end of the band with both hands, rotate toward the center of the body (see figures 6.46 and 6.47).
- Perform 10 to 15 repetitions and switch sides.

Abdominal Crunches

Pettersen braces her torso against a stability ball and focuses on keeping her lower back engaged. Using a band during this core movement adds an enormous amount of stress to the exercise, strengthening both the lower and upper abdominal muscles. Maintaining and developing a strong explosive core not only protects the back but also creates stability and speed in the golf set-up and swing.

- Loop one end of the resistance band around a stable object close to the floor or have another person stand on it.
- Hold the other end of the band with both hands.
- Lie on a stability ball with your back flat on the ball.
- Hold the band above your head with your elbows bent at a 45-degree angle (see figure 6.48).
- Contract your abdominal muscles as you lift toward the ceiling (see figure 6.49).
- Do 10 to 15 repetitions.

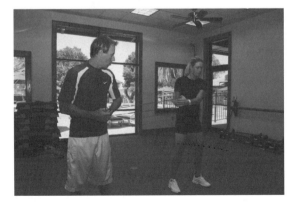

FIGURE 6.46

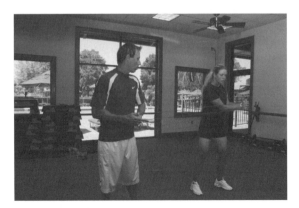

FIGURE 6.47

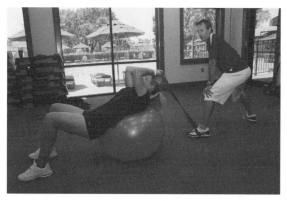

FIGURE 6.48

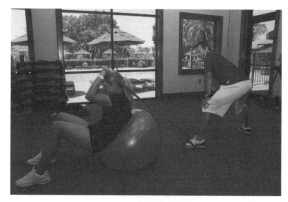

FIGURE 6.49

The Hamstring Stretch

This is an excellent strengthening and stretching exercise for the hamstrings and buttocks. Keeping these muscles loose and flexible is important in maintaining a healthy back.

- Lie flat on the floor on your back.
- Hold one end of the resistance band in each hand.
- Loop the middle of the band around the right foot.
- Raise the right leg straight toward the ceiling (see figure 6.50).
- Hold the stretch on each leg for 10 to 20 seconds and switch legs.

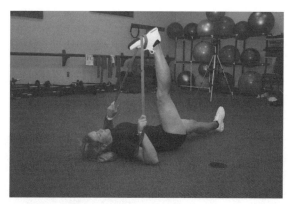

FIGURE 6.50

The Reverse Rotational Core

This is an excellent exercise for warming the core and strengthening the lower back rotational muscles. It is done in the opposite direction of the rotational core exercise.

- Wrap a flex band around a stable object at chest height.
- Grasp the band with your right hand with your palm facing downward.
- Stand with the left leg extended slightly forward to maintain your balance.
- Extend the right arm out in front of you and pull the band toward you until your elbow is aligned with your right side (see figure 6.51).
- Return to the starting position.
- Do 10 to 15 repetitions and switch arms (see figure 6.52).

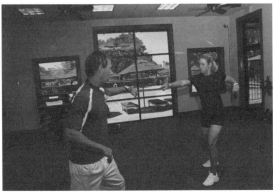

FIGURE 6.51

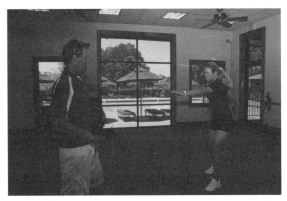

FIGURE 6.52

Bicep Curls

Pettersen performs simple bicep curls using a small resistance band to build balanced muscles in the biceps and triceps, a move that is crucial in maintaining an athletic body. This exercise is also great for building the strength necessary to prevent injuries to the elbows or wrists from the stress of hitting out of the rough.

- Place one end of a resistance band around a stable object or have another person hold it for you.
- Hold the other end of the band with your right hand with your palm facing toward the ceiling.
- Bend your left arm and place your left wrist and hand under your right elbow for support (see figure 6.53).
- Curl your right arm up to 90 degrees (see figure 6.54).
- Release and extend your right arm back to the starting position.
- Perform 10 to 15 repetitions and switch arms.

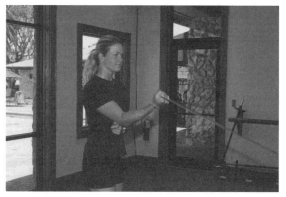

FIGURE 6.53

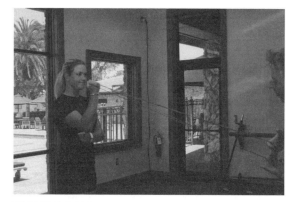

FIGURE 6.54

Triceps Extensions

This exercise warms and strengthens the triceps. Strengthening and developing speed in the triceps are important in creating more speed and explosion throughout the golf swing. Strong triceps are also important in maintaining strong shoulders, elbows, and wrists.

- Place one end of the resistance band around a stable object or have another person hold it for you.
- Hold the other end of the band with your right hand with your right arm bent behind your head and the palm of your hand facing toward the ceiling. Keep the right elbow pulled in close to your head, and place the left hand on your upper right arm for support (see figure 6.55).
- Keep your right arm close to your head as you extend the arm toward the ceiling (see figure 6.56).

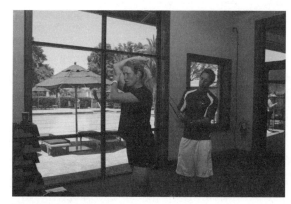

FIGURE 6.55

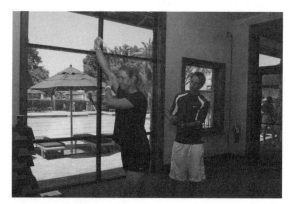

FIGURE 6.56

- Release the arm back to the starting position.
- Do 10 to 15 repetitions and switch arms.

Band Squats

Pettersen uses a medium resistance band to perform leg squats. This is a safe and effective exercise to build strong and explosive legs. A strong and explosive lower body is a major factor in a consistent and powerful swing.

- Using a thin band, step on one end of the band and hold the other end in your hands.
- Hold the other end of the band in your hands and cross your arms in front of your chest.
- Slowly bend both knees until they form a 90-degree angle (see figure 6.57).
- Slowly stand up and return to the start position (see figure 6.58).
- Perform 10 to 15 repetitions.

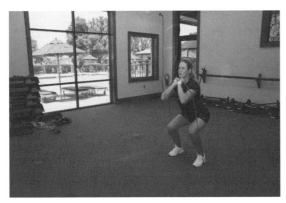

FIGURE 6.57

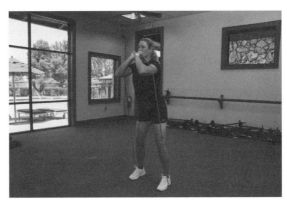

FIGURE 6.58

SUMMARY

Professional golfers know the importance of strength, power, flexibility, core stability, body awareness, and endurance in golf. Most golf professionals train like elite athletes. Although unseen to the general public, professional golfers spend countless hours in the gym conditioning their bodies to perform at the highest possible level. As a recreational golfer, you may not have the time to train like professionals do, but simply incorporating a few exercises into your daily fitness routine two to three times a week can dramatically improve your game and body.

NICK FALDO'S THOUGHTS ON GOLF FITNESS

Golf Fitness Magazine: During your competitive years, was your fitness routine, in your opinion, golf-specific in relation to your health and competitive edge or simply a regime to stay fit? And in hindsight, was your conditioning a prerequisite to your success or something you got into after your golf career began?

Nick Faldo: We were always very conscious of what people would say, like don't lift weights because it will ruin your touch. Obviously they have proved all of that wrong now. Now you can work pretty hard and still maintain touch for the game of golf.

GFM: Do you think it was a prerequisite to your success?

NF: I think it was kind of important. I really don't have to tell you guys, you know, if you are physically strong, you're mentally strong. That has always been important to me. I have always been physically fit. I was a good cyclist. I guess my cardiovascular came from cycling. I used to run. I actually quit running in 1987. I will never forget, I was running up a hill in Sydney, Australia, and the strain on my back, I thought, wow, you know I'm a big guy and this is not for me. Then I became more sport specific for golf, power walking and other things. I've been fortunate that my body is adaptable. I can train in different ways and recover well, so that's probably got something to do with it, too.

GFM: As the number one player in the world and a Ryder Cup champion for a number of years, and assuming your level of fitness was giving you a competitive edge, why do you feel that there wasn't as much attention from other players of the time, about conditioning, as you see on Tour today?

NF: I don't know, I guess we have moved on from it. If you had a good pair of hands, good hand-eye coordination, you could play, but I wanted to play well when I wanted to play well. I always felt like a lot of guys showed up to have a good week, but they couldn't make it happen. Sure it would happen at one stage or another because they were talented golfers. What I was trying to achieve was to be able to play well tomorrow when I really needed it. I did enough that I felt like I had an advantage over those sorts of guys. To be fair, we didn't have all the depth. Mentally I would think, I only have five guys to beat. Now all that has definitely changed. Today the leading guy still knows who they have to beat, but there is still more depth where more players can come through and stay in there, where back in my year, yeah, sure they can come through, but you knew darn well they wouldn't last.

GFM: Do you feel that fitness has reduced your risk of injury and added longevity to your career as a competitive player?

NF: Yes, very much so. I don't know how many millions of golf balls I have hit, and you know my spine is still straight. I started more seriously with balance training. I had a trainer back in 1990 who said I wasn't balanced throughout my body and weak in different areas. That was the first era. My cardiovascular was always good. I always looked after myself. I had a lot of massages and a lot of physiotherapy, and I would go three times a week and she would just go up and down my spine with her thumbs and manipulate my spine, get them all moving. That was very important to me. Now we do so much, playing, training, jumping on airplanes, sitting in cars. It's a brutal life on your neck and back.

GFM: What about Gary Player?

NF: Well, Gary was very inspirational. He did all sorts of stuff, real basic stuff. But the strength of players back then came all from just hitting golf balls. You look at it now (depending solely on hitting golf balls for conditioning), it's very dangerous, very risky.

GFM: If a player only had 10 minutes to warm up before his round, what, in your opinion, would be the most important thing to do in those 10 minutes?

NF: Really simple exercises for your wrists and arms. You can do figure eights with your club. Draw a figure eight with your driver. That warms up your wrists, forearms, and a bit of the rotator cuffs as well. That's quite important. For me, lower back. I might get on the floor and do a few twists here and there just to declunk it, that sort of thing, and then some shoulder stuff, just some rotations of my shoulders to get them warmed up. Also use the golf cart to help you. Stretch your shoulders out some way or another, that's always good to just ease them out a bit.

GFM: What advice would you give to junior golfers about golf-specific fitness and training for success in the sport of golf?

NF: Number one, I think that people assume that because they are young they are supple and flexible, and they are not. They are amazingly tight, these kids, some often having very poor range of motion. I have my own Faldo series, and we have been working on fitness now for most of the 2000s. I have had a variety of different coaches come along to help me to explain it better and try to get them into the routine. The other big one that is so important is stretching before you go to bed. A lot of people think, I will just stretch in the morning. As you know, there is a cool down at night. You have a long day, then you sit and have dinner, and then your lower back tightens up, and then you jump into bed, and it just tightens up even more. So we like to instill a little bit of discipline. We ask them to do something at night before they go to bed, at least the stretching. You probably sleep better as well.

GFM: What are your thoughts on steroid testing for PGA players? Did you ever think that golf would be considered such an athletic sport that this testing would take place among the players?

NF: I think it's because they are getting us ready for the Olympics. I've been out there 30 years and never suspected anything. As golfers we need strength, we need elasticity, we need nerve, and we need touch. If there is a pill or whatever out there that can do all of those (laughs), then send me a few. I can't imagine they are going to find anything. I just hope nobody gets called out for silly obvious things like nasal sprays.

GFM: As much as you travel, is there a "must have" golf fitness aid that you take with you and use on the road, or do you just utilize the gym or in-room routine at the hotel?

NF: I don't need a ton of weights to get in a decent workout. I only need 10- to 15-pound dumbbells and an elliptical trainer for cardio, or, even better, if there is a medicine ball or Swiss ball. That's all I need in my kit. I can create lots of little programs for myself. Whatever a gym has got, I can have a pretty good session.

CHAPTER 7

INJURY AWARENESS

A ROUGH GAME

Last year, golfers suffered approximately 35,000 injuries that required a trip to the emergency room or doctor. Contrary to popular belief, golf is a physical game that requires a lot of swinging, twisting, turning, gripping, bending, and squatting, all of which place stress and strain on the lower back, hips, knees, shoulders, hands, wrists, and elbows. Injuries can also occur if you walk and carry your bag, putting you at higher risk for back, knee, and ankle injuries.

The majority of golf injuries are not usually the result of a single traumatic or fluke accident. They are more frequently the consequence of tissue damage sustained over time from overuse and poor technique. Most golf injuries fall into the general categories of strains, sprains, fractures, and tendonitis. Since the golf swing emphasizes movements on one side of the body more than the other, frequent play can inevitably create muscle imbalances that can lead to injuries.

Golf can take a physical toll on a body. In this chapter, our GFM Advisory Team has assembled the best tips and advice to help you avoid injuries. They also provide information on how to handle what happens if you do get hurt.

THE 10 MOST COMMON GOLF INJURIES

Golf requires a lot of time and effort, not to mention a great deal of skill, mental fortitude, and perseverance if you want to excel at it. The explosive nature of the swing can put a tremendous amount of stress on the body, and a majority of professional golfers have experienced some sort of nagging injury at one time or another during their careers. But you don't have to be a professional to experience some of the most common injuries in golf. Even casual golfers can sustain injuries, but many injuries can be prevented.

Experts in sports medicine note a number of factors that contribute to common golf swing injuries, including the following:

- overuse and too much practice
- poor swing mechanics
- tendency to overswing
- failure to warm up muscles before play
- rotational stress placed on the spine
- incorrect grip and setup
- traumatic force to the body resulting from a poorly executed swing

These factors can lead to the most common injuries.

1. Back Pain

An estimated 75 percent to 85 percent of all Americans will experience some form of back pain during their lifetime, and that number may be higher among golfers. The rotational stresses of the golf swing can place considerable pressure on the spine and muscles. Compound that with the fact that golfers spend four to five hours in a bent-over stance, repeating the same motion hundreds of times. It is no wonder that playing golf can cause minor strains in the back that can easily lead to severe injuries. To keep your back healthy for golf, you should add exercises to your workout routine that stretch and strengthen your back.

2. Tendonitis in the Elbows

Tendonitis (irritation and inflammation of the tendon tissue) is the most common condition affecting the elbow. It is frequently referred to as "tennis elbow," in which case there is an injury to the outer tendon, and "golfer's elbow," when there is an injury to the inner tendon. Interestingly enough, most golfers suffer more from tennis elbow than golfer's elbow. The risk of getting tendonitis increases with age and is higher in people who routinely perform activities that require repetitive movements that increase stress on susceptible tendons, for example, hitting golf balls. In addition, even with less repetition, these types of injuries can be aggravated by improper swing motion.

Treatment focuses on resting the injured tendon to allow healing, decreasing inflammation, promoting muscle strength, and improving swing mechanics. In most patients, tendonitis can be remedied with proper treatment. Failure to get proper treatment can result in a significant amount of pain.

3. Knee Pain

Knee pain can occur from the strain placed on a weak knee when the golfer is trying to stabilize the rotation of the hip axis at the beginning of the swing. Extreme force placed on the knee can result in torn ligaments. Arthritis sufferers may experience more knee problems due to the degenerative nature of the disease, which results in a gradual wearing away of joint cartilage.

Treatment of knee pain depends on the cause of the problem. If you are experiencing symptoms, you should see a doctor. Symptoms include popping, grinding, locking, and swelling of the knee. Stretching, resting, and icing the knee to reduce inflammation can help alleviate symptoms.

4. Rotator Cuff Injuries

Pain may be felt in the shoulder or upper arm at various phases of the golf swing or following play, often during the night and when extending the arms overhead. Injuries to the rotator cuff can be sustained through traumatic force resulting from a poorly executed golf swing, hitting a root or rock, taking a deep divot, or overuse. Golfers can develop tendonitis, bursitis, and tears in the rotator cuff due to the repetitive motion of the golf swing.

Rotator cuff injuries are usually treated with antiinflammatory drugs. In some instances, surgical repair becomes necessary. In these cases, modifications to the golf swing, combined with strength conditioning, can alleviate symptoms and prevent further injury.

5. Wrist Injuries

The repetitive motions of golf and the high speed of the typical golf swing can place the wrists at high risk for injury. Pain and tenderness on top of the wrist, experienced at the top of the backswing and at impact, are common. The most common golf-related wrist injury is tendonitis, or swelling of the tendons responsible for wrist movement. Many wrist injuries and other golf-related injuries can be prevented by performing a preseason and year-round golf-specific conditioning program.

6. Hand and Finger Injuries

As with wrist injuries, the repetitive motions of golf and the high speed of the typical golf swing can place the hands and fingers at high risk for injury. Repetitive blunt trauma or single severe trauma to the fingers can lead to numerous conditions, including tendonitis, broken or deformed bones, and a condition known as hypothenar hammer syndrome (HHS). Learning the proper grip, avoiding long periods of ball bashing, and not hitting balls off of artificial mats can prevent these injuries. (PGA Tour player Aaron Oberholser had a finger injury from playing golf.)

7. Neck Injuries

Neck injuries are common amongst new golfers who are not accustomed to twisting their bodies in different directions. After a few hours of swinging the club and hitting balls, the neck muscles may shorten in spasm and freeze the neck into a painful position. Like most injuries, neck injuries can be prevented by warming up the muscles prior to practice or play, taking frequent breaks while playing or practicing, and slowly working up to longer periods of practice and play. The primary goal of an exercise program for your neck is to strengthen and stretch the shoulders and upper back. (LPGA Tour player Annika Sorenstam had a neck injury during her career.)

8. Foot and Ankle Injuries

When swinging a golf club, the body acts as a whip. Power production starts with the feet pushing against the ground. Each foot moves differently during the swing. The back foot must allow for more pronation during the follow-through than the front foot. Injuries can occur when the golfer loses his or her footing or balance during the swing, while performing the swing with the improper swing mechanics, and when hitting a ball off an uneven surface. Sprains in the ankles, tendonitis in the ankle and foot bones, and inflammation and blisters are common injuries that can be sustained while playing golf. Wearing properly fitted golf shoes and improving swing mechanics are the best ways to prevent foot and ankle injuries.

9. Hip Injuries

The hip joint is very mobile, able to withstand large amounts of loading stresses, but it is particularly vulnerable to injury during golf since the swing involves many pivoting and twisting movements. During the golf swing, the hip is subjected to repeated adduction and flexion/extension forces. This requires a great deal of control throughout the gluteal muscles and adductor muscle complex. These rotational and shear forces cause such ailments as groin strains and lower back injuries.

The hip joint is similar in construction to the shoulder joint or rotator cuff, thus the injuries sustained to the hip are much like the tears that occur to the rotator cuff. Warming up muscles before play is imperative in preventing injury, as is adding flexibility and strength to the muscles that surround the hip joint and socket. (PGA Tour players Jack Nicklaus and Peter Jacobsen had hip replacements.)

10. Sunburn

The skin is the largest organ of the body and the most vulnerable to damage while playing golf. Repeated exposure to the sun can lead to skin damage and even skin cancer. Since golfers typically spend four to five hours exposed to the sun, often during the hottest part of the day, they are prone to sunburns, which can lead to skin injuries.

Prevention is the best defense against the sun. You should always apply sunscreen with an SPF of 15 or higher and reapply often during the round. Wear a hat, sunglasses, and protective clothing if you are going to spend long periods of time in the sun. (PGA Tour players Nick Price and Tom Watson both had skin cancer scares.)

Preventing the most common golf injuries can be done by working on improving swing mechanics, participating in golf-specific conditioning programs, buying properly fitted equipment, avoiding long practice sessions, always performing a warm-up routine before practice and play, and doing golf-specific stretching. Remember these easy pointers to stay in tip-top shape and free from injuries.

CONDITIONING TO PREVENT BACK INJURIES

It is a well-known fact that one of the most common injuries in golf is to the lower back. Research indicates more than half of all golfers will incur a lower back injury at some time during their playing careers. The best way to avoid an injury is to prevent it with proper conditioning and swing mechanics. GFM contributor Rob Price feels that conditioning the midsection, or core, is one of the best and most effective ways to prevent lower back injuries while golfing.

Many golfers tend to neglect the area of the body that fitness experts feel is paramount in athletic performance. The most overlooked, underrated part of the body with respect to competitive golf training is the midsection. The midsection includes the abdominal, oblique, and lower back muscles. The function of strong abs is not just to look good at the beach; a well-trained midsection is the "missing link" to modern golf training and is crucial in taking your athletic ability to the next level and beyond.

Strong abdominal muscles are vital to all golfers for a variety of reasons. Having strong abdominal muscles leads to better balance, faster movements, quicker turns and swings, and increased speed and power. Having a shield of muscle encompassing your trunk also helps in shock absorption and assists in the reduction of lower back injuries. The midsection is a place where power is both created and transferred, allowing you to collectively apply your upper and lower body strength into one harmonious burst of energy.

The absence of a well-trained midsection is not only detrimental to your performance, but it can also negatively affect your health. Lower back injuries plague many golfers worldwide, and the chances of experiencing lower back pain increase as you age. One of the best ways to prevent these types of injuries is to strengthen the muscles of the midsection. Strong core muscles will help drastically reduce the daily stress that is placed on your back muscles and lower lumbar vertebrae. Strengthening your core can also play a major role in injury rehabilitation. Well-trained muscles are more likely to recover faster from injuries, which will reduce chronic pain and soreness.

Unlike other muscles in the body, the midsection is uniquely capable of being trained on a daily basis without experiencing fatigue or overtraining. The midsection should be trained at the onset of every weight-training session. This provides the dual effect of both warming you up by increasing your blood flow and strengthening your abdominal muscles. This can be thought of as killing two birds with one stone.

Working your midsection prior to each weight training session makes your training more efficient by cutting down the time you spend in the gym, while maintaining an equally effective workout.

There are four methods of training the midsection. For the best results, utilize all the techniques. These methods include the following:

1. Keep your upper body stationary while your lower body moves.
2. Keep your lower body stationary while your upper body moves.
3. Use rotational movements.
4. Focus on lower back exercises.

Keeping your upper body stationary while your lower body moves works the lower abdominal muscles, while keeping your lower body stationary while your upper body moves trains the upper abdominal muscles. Focusing on lower back exercises strengthens the lower back. The third method, using rotational movements, is the most beneficial method of training for golfers, because it trains all regions of the midsection and simulates many golf-specific movements. As you swing a golf club, your midsection twists and turns. As you perform rotational movement exercises, think about how they will help you on the course, and concentrate on simulating your golf-specific movements.

The muscles in your midsection are different in nature from the other muscles in your body, and they need to be trained differently to achieve maximum results. To properly train your abdominal muscles, you should do the following:

1. *Use slow movements.* The abdominal muscles are made up of mostly slow-twitch muscle fibers. This type of muscle fiber requires training with slow movements for optimal results.

2. *Train with quantity and consistency.* The abdominal muscles need to be trained for muscular endurance, not muscular strength, which requires numerous repetitions performed daily.

3. *Perform a variety of movements.* Your midsection consists of different areas, each of which requires different exercises for optimum fitness. To train each section, you should perform a variety of exercises. Variety allows you to build, tone, and strengthen each part of the muscles you are training and prevents boredom from setting in at the gym.

An effective method for training your abdominal region is to perform between four and six different midsection exercises during each workout. Perform each exercise slowly and smoothly for one full minute without resting, and rest for 30 seconds between exercises. If you are unable to perform each exercise for one full minute, try working in 30-second increments. You should begin your midsection training with exercises for the lower abdominal muscles, followed by oblique then upper abdominal muscle exercises. This will reduce premature fatigue in the upper abdominal muscles and ensure a holistic approach to your midsection training. Always have a partner or spotter present for motivation and to assist you with proper technique, and never sacrifice quality for quantity.

The results are clearly visible and the correlation is undeniable: A strong, well-trained, and powerful midsection goes hand in hand with increased golf performance. If you are looking to prevent lower back injuries and improve your game, look no further than your stomach.

Improving Posture to Prevent Back Problems

The golf swing is not the most natural moment and is difficult to master. Even if your swing mechanics are absolutely perfect, back injuries can occur. During a golf swing, your body weight is forced through your spine eight times as much as normal as you strike the ball. The stress on your back can be worsened with poor technique, repetition, and poor posture.

Envision the letter "S." Now think of the curve in your lumbar spine (lower back) area. This area resembles the letter "S." With that in mind, think about certain types of incorrect postures or stances, or, better yet, remember the days when your mother used to nag you to stand up straight, hold your shoulders high, suck in your tummy, and sit up straight. Of course the reasons that mom used to nag had nothing to do with your golf swing, but had everything to do with your posture.

Years of incorrect posture and stance can lead to the development of poor posture, referred to as S-posture. This typically means that there is an unbalanced curve in the lumbar spine that often causes pain. Although poor posture is not always the underlying cause of S-posture, this disproportionate curve in the lumbar spine often causes pain, forces the abdominal muscles to relax, and places added pressure on the back.

How does this relate to the golf swing? According to GFM contributor Katherine Roberts, golf fitness expert, when a golfer is unable to create a proper tilt in the lower pelvis region or a proper posterior tilt due to an excessive S-posture, he or she can begin to lose their posture, or "footing," in the golf swing. This can block a certain amount of power that is transferred from the limbs to the core body area. When this happens during the swing, less force is achieved and more injuries occur.

Through three-dimensional motion analysis, we know that more than 90 percent of PGA Tour players have a posterior tilt at the point of impact, helping them generate power from the lower body. If you cannot tuck the pelvis under due to an excessive S-posture, or create a posterior tilt, you prevent your body from generating maximum power.

PREVENTING KNEE INJURIES

Tiger Woods knows the importance of taking care of his knees. In 2008, Woods underwent his third knee surgery since 1994. Since then he has spent a tremendous amount of time rehabbing his left knee. In the two years following his surgery, he managed to come back stronger than ever and win Player of the Year honors.

Woods's surgeries have been on the left knee, the more commonly injured knee for a right-handed golfer. After the lower back, the knee is the most commonly injured joint in golf. Knee pain or injuries can significantly alter swing mechanics and, therefore, result in poor ball placement and higher scores.

There are numerous common knee injuries related to golf. Basic knowledge of knee anatomy is required to understand golf-related injuries. The following is a list of the main anatomical parts of the knee joint, along with a brief description of each part:

- *Bones.* The knee is made up of three bones: the femur, which is the large thigh bone; the tibia, which is the shin bone; and the patella, or the kneecap.
- *Muscles.* The muscles that run across the knee joint are extremely important not only in moving the knee but protecting it and absorbing shock. The main muscles include the quadriceps, or thigh muscle, which extends the knee forward; the hamstring, which sits behind the thigh and bends the knee; and the calf muscle, which pushes the foot down and works as the hamstring's assistant in bending the knee. There are also small muscles that run from the back of the knee into the foot. These muscles work to rotate the knee at the end of straightening to help lock it in position.
- *Ligaments.* There are four main ligaments that support and prevent excess motion at the knee joint. The most famous (or notorious, especially in sports injuries) is the ACL, or the anterior cruciate ligament. Its counterpart is the PCL, or posterior cruciate ligament. These two ligaments run between the femur and tibia under the

patella and help prevent excess forward or backward movement of the knee. The MCL, or medial collateral ligament, is a wide ligament that runs on the inside of the knee connecting the femur and tibia. The forth ligament, the LCL (lateral collateral ligament), is on the outside of the knee joint. These ligaments are important in side-to-side movements.

- *Cartilage.* Between the femur and tibia sit two C-shaped menisci, or cartilage. This cartilage acts to distribute shock between the lower and upper leg and helps guide the motion at the knee.

Now that we have a basic understanding of knee anatomy, let's discuss common injuries or problems associated with the knee. The following is a list of common knee pathologies:

- *Osteoarthritis.* Osteoarthritis is the most common knee problem and the second leading cause of disability in Americans over the age of 65. This pathology is the wear and tear of joints and is often the result of poor mechanics. This can be due to tight and/or weak muscles, previous injuries to the joint, and overuse of the joint. Signs and symptoms of osteoarthritis include stiffness and swelling that is worse in the morning or after resting and improves slightly with activity.

- *Condromalacia.* Condromalacia is the wear and tear or softening of the undersurface of the kneecap. Similar to osteoarthritis, condromalacia can be the result of poor mechanics at the knee joint. Dull pain and/or grinding are often felt under the kneecap, and the pain is worsened upon climbing hills or stairs.

- *Torn ligaments.* Strains or tears (partial or full) are common with activities that involve sudden starts, stops, and pivoting. Such ligament injuries as ACL tears are often seen in basketball, soccer, and football. With a ligament injury, a loud pop is often heard. There may or may not be pain associated with a full ligament tear.

- *Meniscal injuries.* The meniscus is often injured with twisting or pivot motions. Because the menisci lack good blood supply, they do not heal as most other tissues do. Meniscal injuries often cause clicking and catching sensations in the knee, especially when squatting or bending.

- *Tendonitis.* Tendons often become inflamed and irritated due to overuse or improper use of muscles. This affliction is especially common in those just starting out a new activity or when changing form without allowing enough time for rest.

There are various causes of knee problems related to golf. Many of these problems have a direct correlation to the amount of rotation required throughout the body during the backswing and follow-through. For a right-handed golfer, a significant amount of torque and valgus stress (stress to the inside of the knee) is generated at the left knee. The knees must stay flexed during the backswing to absorb some of the rotational stress of the swing.

For the many golfers who have tight back muscles and joints, one of the ways to attempt to generate more turn in the backswing is to place more stress on the knee. This often leads to injuries to the medial (inside) meniscus. There are also many golfers with tight hip muscles, which changes the joint alignment at the knee. This again places more stress on the knee, making it more susceptible to injury.

Another possible cause of or contributor to knee pain is poor-fitting or poor-supporting shoes. Golf shoes that do not provide enough arch support can lead to a pronated foot position (flattened arch), which places the knee in a rotated position. During the course of walking 18 holes or up and down hills and through sand traps, this foot and knee position can lead to a significant amount of knee pain.

The knee is not designed to execute the rotation and side-to-side movements required by the golf swing. Because of this, precautions should be taken to ensure that extra stress is not placed on the knees. One of the best measures is to ensure that the muscles in the hips, lower back, and middle back are flexible. By allowing full rotation to occur through the hips and back, stress is evenly distributed throughout the knee, and injury will not occur. It is also important to make sure that the three main muscles surrounding the knee joint are strong. By making certain that these three main muscles are strong and the hips and back are flexible, the knee joint is afforded maximal protection against injury. Your physical therapist or personal trainer can help you with flexibility and strengthening exercises to target these areas to decrease the stress on your knees.

If you are recovering from a knee injury, there are some tips for your preliminary return to playing golf. Start by practicing at the driving range several weeks prior to playing your first round of 18 holes. When you first start to practice, start by hitting wedges and short irons. Begin your practice session by making short swings, working toward full swings and eventually into longer irons and the driver.

If you have had surgery, you should wear spikeless shoes upon your return to golf. These shoes should have good arch support to prevent knee rotation. There are many specialty golf shoe and sneaker stores that can fit you with arch support for your sneakers and golf shoes. In some cases, custom-made orthotics from your health care professional may be required to provide optimal foot positioning. Orthotics can help the knee and decrease strain on the hips and back. Knee braces should only be worn for temporary support after a mild injury and should not be worn on a long-term basis. Any brace that is worn for a lengthy period of time may cause the body to rely on that extra support and can actually weaken or suppress the structural support system.

As always, any injury that prevents you from playing or walking normally or lasts longer than a few days needs to be examined by your health care professional. Playing through a knee injury can worsen the injury and lengthen the recovery time needed to get back on the course. Strong knees and flexible back muscles help ensure smooth movement through the entire backswing and follow-through, helping your shots go straighter and longer.

GETTING A GRIP ON WRIST INJURIES

A wrist injury can be devastating for a professional golfer. Phil Mickelson had to withdraw from several tournaments in 2007 because of a lingering left wrist injury sustained playing a practice round at Oakmont CC, the site of the 2007 US Open. The left-hander failed to contend seriously in any of the four major championships that year because of his nagging wrist.

Wrist injuries are common among golfers and normally occur at the moment of impact between the club and the ball. Teen golf sensation Michelle Wie also had a disappointing year in 2007 on the LPGA Tour because of a similar injury to her right wrist. Wie hit a shot off a cart path during the women's Samsung World Championship in 2006, and the injury caused her to withdraw from several tournaments and led to a disappointing year in 2007.

Because the grip is the body's sole connection to the golf club, wrist action is a crucial part of the swing. The repetitive motions of golf and the high speed of the typical golf swing place wrists at high risk for injury. Let's look at symptoms one might experience with an injured wrist, which include the following:

- hot sensations in the wrist
- swelling of the wrist

- stiffness of the wrist
- pain and discomfort in the wrist during such normal movements as opening jars, turning a door handle, carrying luggage, or shaking hands
- small lumps on the back of the wrist commonly known as ganglions
- pressure on the top of the wrist that causes severe pain
- weakness in the wrist and hand that increases with time
- severe pain in the wrist and hand that leads to use of the nondominant wrist and hand
- increased apprehension and anxiety when using the hand and wrist
- quitting on golf shots at impact due to increased pain and sensitivity

If you are experiencing any of these symptoms before, during, or after your golf game, the next step is to get a proper diagnosis from your physician, as this area of the body is very complex. Many of the structures that are damaged in wrist injuries cannot be seen on a plain x-ray. An MRI is essential in locating the injury and determining whether it is an injury to the tendons, bone, ligaments, nerves, joints, and so forth. You must have a physician's diagnosis to properly treat your symptoms and get the proper rehabilitation.

Many golfers that suffer from wrist injuries have experienced a past injury to the wrist or forearm. These golfers are extremely likely to suffer a recurrence of wrist pain. Wrist injuries that go untreated can lead to more serious permanent damage in the underlying structure of the wrist, for example, the joint discs or ligaments.

After you have confirmed your diagnosis, there are several ways in which you and your physical therapist or physician can work together to rehabilitate your injury. The following are some of the ways in which wrist injuries are commonly treated after a proper diagnosis has been made:

- Rest and apply ice.
- Perform muscular strengthening and flexibility exercises.
- Formulate a short, practical pregame warm-up routine.
- Adjust your golf swing to meet your physical capacities and consider your limitations through properly supervised golf lessons.
- Select the proper golf equipment and consider the environmental conditions.
- Participate in ongoing physical therapy with your therapist, physician, and instructor to diagnose, treat, and repair the injury.

Now that we have evaluated your symptoms and discussed some of the less complex treatments for caring for wrist injuries, the question of how the injury happened still exists. The following is a detailed list of how most golf-related wrist injuries occur:

- *Poor neck posture and muscle control.* The body as a system is quite versatile in adjusting to adverse situations. Poor posture and lack of muscle control can easily lead to compensations in the golf swing. Instead of using large muscle groups to create power in the swing, someone with poor neck posture and muscle control may compensate by flicking the wrists and trying to help the ball up in the air, putting strain on the smaller muscles in the hands and wrists.

- *Prolonged sitting followed by excessive practice ball bashing.* Prolonged periods of inactivity followed by lengthy periods of physical activity, like ball striking, make you more prone to injury. Warming up and cooling down and consistent moderate activity are important in reducing the risk of muscle and joint injuries, especially to the smaller muscles of the wrists.

- *Overuse of the small muscle groups.* Straining the small muscle groups causes fatigue. As with poor neck posture and weak muscle control, if you have weak shoulders, you tend to use other muscles to compensate for the lack of strength and control. If the body cannot stabilize during a swing, other parts of the body, for example, the wrists, will be overused and injured.

- *Overcocking the wrists.* All good players have one position in the golf swing that's similar despite their very different swings. This position is impact. Good players retain their wrist cock through the hitting area so that their left wrist is bowed and the right wrist flexed (for right-handed golfers) and both hands are slightly in front of the golf ball at the strike.

- High-handicappers tend to do the opposite at impact. Instead of a late hit, they execute what is known as an early release. They scoop the ball at impact because they lose the lag too early in the downswing. Instead of having a bowed left wrist and their hands ahead of the ball at impact, they have a collapsed left wrist and their hands behind the ball. As such, they put a tremendous amount of pressure on the muscles and tendons of the wrists, which can lead to injury. A player may damage his or her left wrist in an attempt to overdo the bowed left wrist at impact. Learning the correct mechanics can help prevent injuries.

- *Poor swing technique.* A steep angle of attack on the ball at impact causes the leading wrist to dorsiflex, or extend. As this happens, the elbow's flexor muscles stretch excessively. If the golfer hits the ground first (a fat shot), at the moment of impact, the trauma may damage the tendons and muscles. Many high-handicappers decelerate at the moment of impact to help the ball up in the air. This maneuver puts a tremendous amount of strain on tendons. The result is the lead arm looking like a chicken wing and a weak golf shot.

- *Excessive ball bashing, resulting in poor technique and wrist fatigue and eventual injury of the wrist.* Generally, the more often you play, the higher your risk of injury. Golfers who spend more than six hours per week playing golf are at an increased risk for overuse injuries. Practice habits contribute significantly. The onset of club championships or a New Year's resolution to improve your game may increase your predisposition to injury.

- *Playing on poor quality driving range mats or in heavy rough, causing direct trauma.* Hitting balls off of rubber mats or hard surfaces increases the likelihood of a wrist injury. The constant pounding on the wrists combined with poor swing technique can cause a strain on the muscles. Improper swing technique dramatically increases the risk of injury. Golfers who swing correctly and smoothly are less likely to hurt themselves.

- Hitting out of heavy rough or buried lies or making contact with immovable surfaces (tree roots and rocks) may also lead to injury. Phil Mickelson's wrist injury was caused by hitting a shot out of the rough during a practice round for the US Open. As the clubhead approaches impact, the grass wraps around the head and stops it from sliding through the grass. This can jolt the wrist into an unnatural position.

- *Poor predisposing power and functional grip.* It is imperative that golfers maintain good muscle function in their hands. What happens at the point of impact determines the trajectory of the golf ball, that is, the direction and distance the ball flies. The interaction between the clubface and ball largely depends upon the strength of the wrists. If a golfer has weak grip strength, he or she is at greater risk of injury.

■ **Seniors Tee**
ARTHRITIS PREVENTION ON AND OFF OF THE COURSE

Although commonly thought of as a disease that affects the elderly, arthritis can strike anyone, regardless of race, age, or sex. According to the Arthritis Foundation and the Centers for Disease Control and Prevention, arthritis is one of the most common causes of disability in the United States. It is projected that there will be a 50 percent increase in arthritis over the next 25 years as Baby Boomers age. Although there are many types of arthritis, the most common is osteoarthritis. This type of arthritis is known for the wear and tear it causes on cartilage and joint surfaces. There are many ways to help manage arthritis, including exercise and medication that may be prescribed by your physician. Let's take a look at managing arthritis from the standpoint of preventing or delaying the effects that may alter your golf game.

The four main factors that influence the likelihood of getting arthritis include age, genetics, weight, and injury or overuse of a joint. Two of the four factors cannot be changed. There is no Fountain of Youth, and we cannot yet change our genetic makeup; however, the other two factors, the two most important factors, can be influenced by small changes in your daily life.

The effect that weight has on our joints is often underestimated. Each extra pound that we carry has a multiple-fold effect on our joints, especially the knees. Maintaining the appropriate weight for your body type is essential for healthy joints. For arthritis sufferers, a combination of specifically designed aquatic exercise classes for arthritis or weight loss, as well as exercise programs, can protect the joints. Your physician, physical therapist, nutritionist, personal trainer, or other specialist can help design a program for exercise and nutrition that will minimize obesity as a risk factor for arthritis. There are also many online resources that provide this same information.

The second risk factor that can be controlled, or at least managed, is injury to or overuse of joints. Research suggests that arthritis is due in part to poor early joint care and misuse. Physical therapists are specially trained to assess the quantity and quality of movement in the joints. There are hands-on techniques that they can perform on each joint to improve this movement to avoid placing extra stress on the joint and cartilage and decrease the risk for arthritis in that joint. A joint will respond better to these techniques early in the healing stage; however, there is the potential for improvement even years after an injury. If you suspect that you have had such an injury, see your physician for a referral to a physical therapist who can perform a thorough joint evaluation. Early joint care will ensure that you are playing pain-free golf long into retirement.

ELBOW OVERUSE INJURIES

Tennis and golfer's elbow are often the result of "overuse injuries." Overuse injuries are the cumulative effect of many tiny injuries caused by stress or strain on body tissue. This type of injury can occur suddenly but often develops slowly over time. Each time we use our body to perform a movement, we create these microscopic injuries, or tears, in the muscles, tendons (which connect muscles to bones), ligaments (which connect bones to bones), and even the bones themselves. Our bodies become stronger by responding to these injuries by building stronger muscles, tendons, ligaments, and bones. This is what happens each time we exercise.

Overuse injuries occur when we exceed our body's ability to rebuild tissue as fast as we damage it. This causes inflammation and can limit our body's ability to heal itself. Over time, this inflammation can become chronic and limit strength and range of motion. It can also be very painful. Overuse injuries are common in areas where any one motion is repeated, for example, running, playing tennis, using a computer keyboard, or lifting something overhead.

Tennis Elbow versus Golfer's Elbow

Tennis elbow and or golfer's elbow both involve inflammation of the tendons where they attach to the bony areas of the elbow. Tennis elbow, or lateral epicondylitis, affects the tendons on the outside of the elbow. The opposite of this is golfer's elbow, or medial epicondylitis, which affects the tendons on the inside of the elbow. Any type of elbow pain is often referred to as "tennis elbow" simply due to popularity of the term. Tennis elbow and golfer's elbow are actually misnomers, as there are many causes and activities related to medial and lateral epicondylitis.

As the muscles of the forearm work to move the wrist and hand, they contract and pull on the bony areas on the inside or outside of the elbow. Repeated tugging on these muscles causes tiny tears in the muscles and tendons. If we injure the tissue faster than our bodies can repair it, the result is pain, tenderness, inflammation, decreased strength, and decreased range of motion at the elbow and wrist. It may be difficult to fully bend or straighten the elbow, turn the forearm (e.g., turning a key in a door or ignition of a car), type, or grip items (e.g., raising a cup of coffee or pulling open a door).

True tennis elbow is often caused by improper grip of the tennis racket, repeated use of a backhand swing, faulty swing mechanics, arm weakness, poor warm-up or cool-down techniques, or any combination of these. The muscles that attach to the outside of the elbow draw the wrist backward, so any activity that mimics that motion may also contribute to elbow pain. With golfer's elbow the muscles on the inside of the elbow work to draw the wrist forward, grip the golf club, or make a fist. Like tennis elbow, golfer's elbow can be caused by faulty swing mechanics, tight or improper club grip, increased wrist action during the golf swing, or any other action that causes the wrist to be flexed forward.

There are many other causes of elbow pain. Tennis elbow or golfer's elbow can easily be caused by nonsport activities. Repeated use of a keyboard, especially with a poor computer setup, is one of the most common nonsport-related causes of tennis elbow. Repeated gripping activities like using a screwdriver or hammer can also cause elbow pain due to the strain placed on the muscles of the wrist and elbow.

Elbow pain can also be caused by many other factors not directly related to the elbow. Physical therapists look beyond the elbow and wrist to the neck, the shoulder, and posture as potential sources of elbow pain. Degeneration in the neck leading to pressure on the nerves going into the arm, poor rotator cuff strength, and a slouched posture are examples of other causes that may mimic tennis or golfer's elbow.

If you have elbow pain, there are several ways to treat it. The sooner you treat the pain, the more likely you are to have better and quicker results. The first step is to rest the arm. Stop doing the activity that you think is most bothering your elbow. If you are a professional athlete or someone who uses the computer keyboard at work, try to modify or change the activity so that it places less stress on your elbow.

The second step is to ice the area that hurts. Use a gel ice pack or ice cubes on the painful area for 10 to 15 minutes several times per day. You may want to take over-the-counter pain relievers or such anti-inflammatory medicines as Advil, Motrin, or Aleve. Consult your health care professional before starting any medications. Compression wraps are also available at drugstores to help distribute the load on the elbow.

If these options are not helpful, consult your physician, physical therapist, or occupational therapist. Your physician may prescribe medications or recommend a cortisone injection. Your physical or occupational therapist will show you specific stretches and strengthening exercises and examine you for other potential causes of the pain.

The most important factor in long-term success of reducing or preventing elbow pain is to address the factor that originally placed the added stress on the elbow. If you are a golfer, consult your coach on the mechanics of your swing and the equipment you are using. If you are

STAY MENTALLY AND PHYSICALLY ACTIVE TO PREVENT DISEASE AND STAY ALERT

In 2005, Ohio State University researchers reported that older people who exercised regularly were more likely to maintain the mental acuity required to do such everyday tasks as following a recipe or keeping track of the pills they take. The important thing is to get into the habit of doing physical and mental exercises when you are young so that these practices are already ingrained in you as you get older.

If golf is your sport, starting a golf-specific exercise program that includes strength training and flexibility is the perfect way to help maintain the body throughout your later years. Incorporating puzzles, games, and crossword activities are excellent ways to maintain your mental acuity. All it takes is 30 minutes per day.

Regular exercise for at least 30 minutes a day is a great way to diminish the negative effects of aging. Aerobic exercise helps get the blood cruising through your system, carrying oxygen and glucose, two substances the brain needs to function, to your brain. Regular exercise also encourages the brain to produce more of the molecules that help protect and produce the brain's neurons. Starting a golf-specific exercise program can not only help your game, it may also help you prevent such afflictions as heart disease, osteoporosis, diabetes, obesity, and even Alzheimer's.

experiencing elbow pain related to your job or daily activities, a physical or occupational therapist will look at the ergonomics to ensure the optimal setup.

NECK PAIN: IS IT SOMETHING YOU SHOULD WORRY ABOUT?

It is a beautiful day at your favorite course. Your ball is lying deep, but your hard swing doesn't quite flow through, and *bam*! You feel a twinge in your neck. The next morning your neck is stiff, aching, and you can't turn your head. Now what? For most of us, such an ailment will heal itself with the best medicine of all, time. Throw in some anti-inflammatory medicines, rest, passive range of motion, and perhaps some massage, physical therapy, and corticosteroid treatment prescribed by your physician, and in most cases there are no further problems.

In other cases, there are circumstances that require early evaluation that should not be ignored. You may be suffering from a herniated disc in your neck, and it is important not to miss any of the important clues that may lead you to miss out on golf or any other of life's joyful activities because of damage to the spinal cord or a nerve.

But don't panic. Most herniated discs are not severe, and 90 percent of them do not require intervention; however, it is important to understand which herniations are severe enough to cause permanent injury. There are instances where injury to a nerve or the spinal cord can cause lasting damage. What are the signs of a potential problem, and what should you do about it?

There are several easily recognized symptoms of spinal cord and nerve involvement that indicate the need to seek immediate attention from your physician. Any neck pain associated with numbness of the hands or arms; electrical shocks going down your arms or spine; and weakness in the pushing, pulling, and grasping movements of your wrists are major worries and should prompt attention. Pain or weakness while walking and lack of coordination or difficulty picking things up or manipulating them with your fingers may be further clues to subtle and sometimes confusing nerve damage.

If you have any of these symptoms, see your physician so he or she can determine further treatment, which could involve an MRI of the cervical spine. In the hands of a spine expert, this noninvasive, simple test can easily tell whether you are at risk for further spinal cord or nerve injury.

If an MRI shows an injury, there is good news for treatment. Artificial discs for the cervical spine have recently become available in the United States and abroad that can allow surgical repair of a herniated disc. Without the need for spinal fusion and with a quick and rapid recovery time, many people are back to their normal regimen within several weeks of surgery, even playing golf. Only spine experts can properly evaluate you for this potential treatment, should you be one of the few who has neurological symptoms or fails to improve in time.

If you are exhibiting neurological symptoms, it is a big mistake to assume anything, to have your condition treated with manipulation or traction, or to even ignore it without proper evaluation. We play golf to develop our skills, overcome our adversities, strengthen our weaknesses, and use our good common sense. Since golf is the ultimate game of common sense, we do not want to miss the opportunity to take care of a problem before it takes care of us. While most neck pain and stiffness will get better in a few days, we need to play smart and safe and know the difference when it counts.

SUMMARY

Playing golf puts a lot of strain on the body. It's no surprise that so many golfers experience some sort of injury during their playing careers. To maintain a healthy, powerful golf swing and reduce the risk of injury, it is essential to warm up before play; practice; and follow a golf-specific fitness plan that includes strength, flexibility, and endurance training.

PART
II

THE MIND,
HEALTH,
AND
WELLNESS

CHAPTER 8

PILATES AND YOGA FOR GOLF

Although yoga and Pilates have been in the mainstream of general fitness for several years, golfers are just starting to consider how these two disciplines can help improve their golf games. Such PGA Tour players as Camilo Villegas and Vijay Singh have been practicing either yoga or Pilates for years with dramatic results.

We have all heard how these two types of low-impact exercises are good for our general physical well-being. Yoga has long been considered a therapeutic exercise that incorporates the mind and body, and Pilates heightens our body awareness, which in turn improves overall agility, flexibility, and strength. But how can these two disciplines be beneficial to our golf game, and what is the difference between the two?

The word *yoga* means "union" or "harmony." Yoga is a healing system of theory and practice. It is a combination of breathing exercises, physical postures, and meditation that has been practiced for more than 5,000 years. It focuses on making you aware of your body's posture, alignment, and patterns of movement to make the body more flexible and help you relax. Yoga movements are mostly performed on a special mat with the aid of various props. The body's own weight is used for resistance, and a great deal of focus is accorded to the flow from one posture into the other.

Pilates is a discipline system that was developed in the early twentieth century in Germany by Joseph Pilates to help wounded soldiers in the recovery process. It was later used to help ballet dancers recover from their injuries. It is based on the idea that once you strengthen your core, everything else follows. The moves focus on the abdomen, or core, which is exceptionally beneficial to anyone looking to improve their golf swing. Pilates can be practiced free standing or on a machine called a "reformer."

How can yoga or Pilates help you improve your golf swing? We all know that developing overall body strength with flexibility, stability, balance, posture, alignment, and coordination are important for a biomechanically correct golf swing. These can all be developed and improved by practicing either yoga or Pilates. "A total of 53 percent of male and 45 percent of female golfers suffer from back pain. At any given time, 30 percent of all professional golfers are injured," says Katherine Roberts, GFM contributor and author of *Yoga for Golfers* and *Swing Flaws and Fitness Fixes*. By following a carefully designed program like the one detailed in *Yoga for Golfers*, the risk of injury can be reduced." A golfer already suffering from an injury can also have much greater success returning to the game if he or she addresses the underlying cause of the problem," adds Roberts.

"Pilates is a body conditioning routine that seeks to build flexibility, strength, endurance, and coordination without adding muscle bulk," says Laura Cippola, a certified fitness trainer, sports performance nutrition specialist, GFM contributor, and founder of Golf Fitness International. "In addition, Pilates increases circulation and helps to sculpt the body and strengthen the body's core, or 'powerhouse.' Pilates exercises run many parallels with the game of golf itself: Both require concentration, control, precision, and a good foundation," adds Cippola.

This chapter provides both yoga and Pilates exercises and routines designed specifically by our GFM contributing experts to help improve your flexibility, strength, endurance, breathing, coordination, and even mental acuity for a better golf swing and game.

PREROUND PILATES: A SOUND INVESTMENT FOR YOUR GOLF GAME

Golfers spend millions of dollars on equipment and lessons in the search for that "edge" without considering that their body is their best equipment. This simple 10-minute course-friendly routine could be the best investment you make for this physically and mentally demanding sport. Give it a try. All you have to lose are aches, pains, and strokes off your game.

Since approximately 60 percent of amateur golfers experience some sort of injury while playing, and golf-related injuries force many professional golfers into retirement, a pregame routine of simple movements is an effective way to both combat injury and improve your game. This often-overlooked component of a golfer's game provides a foundation for the techniques required for a successful round.

A few hastily done twists may get the circulation going, but it is foolish to believe that this effort is sufficient for the demands of golf. It is important to not let the serenity of the golf game overshadow its physical demands and the player's potential for injury. Preparing your body for the exertion required by the game does not have to be complicated or time consuming. Studies show that just 10 minutes of stretching before you tee off can d̶͞

Pilates is a safe an
golfer seeing the bene
can do Pilates, regardl
sional status, injury or
your game provides the

- warms up the spina
  of motion, stabilize
  resulting in a more
- improves postural
  through and take si
  injuries
- increases flexibility a
  motion in the lower
- strengthens the hand
  allowing for more eff
- fosters increased endu
  level of play and prev
- improves concentrati
  consistent level of play
- prevents injury

Breathing is an integr
keeps oxygen circulating, ir
erly, it strengthens the deep
back. While performing the
the abdominal muscles en
and exhaling. Posture is also
toward the ceiling, engaging
into your back pockets, and ̶ ̶ ̶ ̶ your chin slightly as if there were a string from the center of your head to the ceiling.

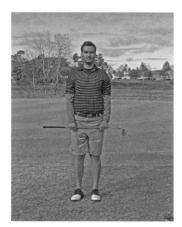

FIGURE 8.1

The game of golf incorporates extensive action from the muscles. The golf swing is not a natural movement. The body is externally and internally rotating, adducting, abducting, flexing, stabilizing, and extending. The benefits of adding 10 minutes to your round will not only increase your longevity in playing the game, it will shave strokes off your score and enable you to get out of bed the next morning with fewer aches and pains.

Roll Downs

Target: spine and hamstrings muscles
Benefit: hamstring flexibility to aid in holding proper spine angle and spine flexibility to increase turning potential for a bigger swing

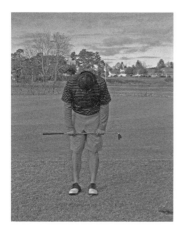

FIGURE 8.2

- Stand tall with your arms relaxed and hold a club in front of you horizontally with both hands (see figure 8.1).
- Inhale and pull your stomach toward your spine.
- Drop your chin to your chest and exhale.
- Roll your back down toward your feet one vertebra at a time while keeping the club close to your legs. Let the weight of your head and arms pull you down into a comfortable stretch (see figure 8.2).
- At the bottom of the stretch, inhale deeply, keeping stomach pulled up and in.
- Exhale as you roll slowly back up. Visualize gently pressing each vertebra against a wall as you move back into a standing position.
- Repeat the move three times.

Side Bends

Target: spine and oblique muscles
Benefit: lateral spine mobility and increased hip turn

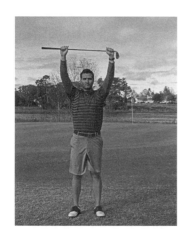

FIGURE 8.3

- Stand tall and hold a club horizontally with both hands.
- Inhale and extend your arms overhead, reaching toward the ceiling (see figure 8.3).
- Exhale and draw your shoulders away from your ears and reach up and over to one side. Imagine that you are hugging a beach ball against your side.
- Inhale and reach out even further (see figure 8.4).
- Exhale as you move back into a standing position.
- Repeat the move three times on each side.

The Weight Shift

Target: core stability
   Benefit: strengthens the entire system for balance

- Stand tall with your feet hip distance apart and eyes facing forward.
- Shift all your weight onto your left leg, keeping it straight but not locked.
- Inhale and then exhale as you lift your right leg and bend the right knee until the knee is aligned with your hip (see figure 8.5).
- Hold for 15 seconds.
- Inhale as you lower the right foot onto the ground.
- Repeat the move three times on each leg.

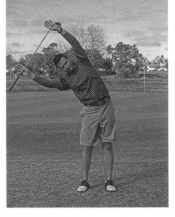

FIGURE 8.4

Arm Circles

Target: Rotator cuff
   Benefit: prepares rotator cuff muscles for the golf swing and increases shoulder turn

- Stand tall with your arms at your sides and your torso still.
- Draw a full circle with your arms by extending them in front of your body, reaching toward the ceiling, and rolling them behind your back (see figures 8.6 and 8.7). Do not turn your torso to make larger circles.
- Repeat the move slowly five times and then reverse the direction.

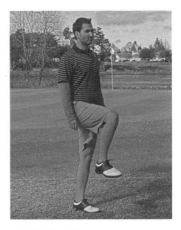

FIGURE 8.5

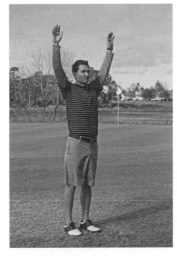

FIGURE 8.6

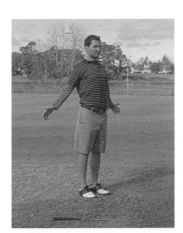

FIGURE 8.7

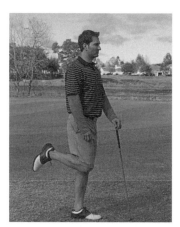

FIGURE 8.8

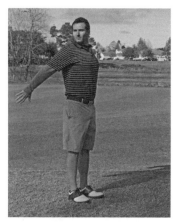

FIGURE 8.9

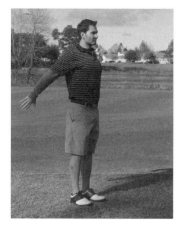

FIGURE 8.10

Standing Leg Flexion

Target: knee and hamstring muscles
  Benefit: knee joint stability

- Stand tall and hold the club in the left hand, resting it on the ground for stability, if necessary.
- Bend the right knee until it forms a 90-degree angle, slowly bringing your heel toward your buttocks (see figure 8.8). Keep your stomach tucked up and in and your tailbone tucked slightly under.
- Hold for 10 seconds and then lower the leg with control.
- Repeat the move three times on each leg.

Chest Expansion

Target: chest
  Benefit: scapular stability and postural strength

- Stand tall with your heels together and toes fist width apart.
- Lift your arms straight out in front of you to shoulder height with your palms facing down.
- Inhale as you pull your stomach up and in.
- Exhale and lower your arms toward the floor and then raise them behind your back. Squeeze the shoulder blades together and open into the chest.
- Inhale and look to the right (see figure 8.9).
- Exhale as you return to the center (see figure 8.10).
- Repeat the move three times on each side.

USING YOGA TO CURE YOUR COMMON SWING FLAWS

Are you a golfer who is plagued by swing flaws that you cannot conquer, regardless of the amount of time and money you spend on lessons and the latest technology? If you have discovered that you have a physical limitation that is causing one or more swing flaws, you may be your own answer to your problems.

Yoga, one of the world's oldest fitness tools, is now being embraced by golfers as a way to improve fitness both on and off of the course. "Certain yoga positions can help golfers correct and eliminate specific swing flaws," says Katherine Roberts, GFM contributor, fitness expert,

REAL GOLFERS DO PILATES

Just as golfers are now being seen as "real" athletes, both professional and amateur athletes in all sports are accepting Pilates as "real" exercise. Professional baseball, basketball, and football stars, and, of course, such professional golfers as Camilo Villegas, are discovering the power of Pilates. The new breed of young golfer understands that fitness is a key component of playing the game, but to many golfers, "getting in shape" equates to lifting weights. Weight lifting builds short, bulky muscles. Pilates builds long, lean muscles. These strong yet flexible muscles give golfers the optimal biomechanics for the swing.

Camilo Villegas is fit and strong, but it is his flexibility that differentiates him from the pack. While Villegas's ultra-flexible Spiderman pose for reading the green is popular with the gallery, it is the amount of turn he gets that is most impressive. In both the backswing and follow-through, the entire upper body, including the shoulders, upper back, and chest, must be able to turn freely and smoothly. If there is any restriction, the golfer will compensate, creating risk of injury. The amount of turn Villegas creates with his flexible upper body is what gives him the fast clubhead speed for those long drives we all envy. Camilo has been doing Pilates since his college days at the University of Florida and says the program gives him "maximum flexibility and core strength."

In a 2003 *USA Today* interview, star pitcher Curt Schilling sums up a typical response from men to Pilates exercise. "The first three weeks, I was really disappointed," says Schilling. "I wasn't sweating. I wasn't winded, which is what I associate with true exercise. Then in the fourth week I started to understand the Pilates terminology, the idea of working from your center. By the third month, I was more powerful and flexible than ever before. And I'd lost 15 pounds."[1]

This common response is due to several factors. First, Pilates is a technique for moving in a way that is efficient, natural, and pain-free. It is not a group of special exercises but rather how we should move in every aspect of life. Consequently, Pilates students must relearn how to move properly. Pilates exercises for beginners may seem easy as you are developing the building blocks for the more difficult work. Just as you must master the fundamentals of golf, perfecting these beginner exercises and learning the Pilates techniques is essential. You will eventually be able to move on to the more difficult exercises. Pilates will not make you sore because Pilates does not work the muscles to exhaustion. Pilates is about performing fewer, more precise, and controlled perfect movements rather than endlessly exhausting and mindless exercises.

It is important to remember that "muscling through" the exercises without really applying the Pilates principles will not give you the desired results. Many students mistakenly go right to intermediate or advanced Pilates workouts without mastering the beginner techniques.

and Golf Channel contributor. "Lack of mobility and stability in the hips are the culprit behind three of the most common swing flaws that golfers face, and practicing yoga may help you conquer these flaws," she continues. According to Roberts, three of the most common swing flaws golfers face are:

1. *Sway.* Sway occurs in the golf swing when the lower body leans away from the target on the backswing, placing excessive weight on the outside of the back foot and impairing balance. The excessive lower body motion inhibits the correct weight shift on the downswing and follow-through.

2. *Coming over the top.* Coming over the top refers to the motion of the downswing when a player swings the club shaft in a circular motion away from the body as the transition is made from the top of the backswing to the start of the downswing.

3. *Loss of posture.* Loss of posture is when a player loses the body angle established at setup during the swing motion. It is a common culprit of lower back stress and injuries.

These swing flaws are often caused by lack of mobility and stability in the hips. Working on these issues by simply doing functional and movement drills may not permanently cure you of swing flaws. There are many additional components you should consider when trying to alleviate the problem, including proper swing mechanics, timing, and sequencing. But increasing flexibility and strength in the hips should be the first step.

For the majority of golfers, starting with a simple, effective fitness program is the key to a better golf swing, no matter what the swing flaw. Strength and flexibility in the hips supports the loading or harnessing of strength and power in the swing and plays an essential role in the acceleration phase of the swing. The ability to access power for more distance, initiate your lower body in the proper sequence to help you stop coming over the top, and rotate your hips around a stable right side is essential for overcoming sway. In addition, lower back pain often originates from improper hip function, shortened hip flexors and adductors, core instability, and weak gluteal muscles. Adding yoga to your fitness routine can allow you to do the following for a better golf game:

- improve your posture at the address position
- generate more power at impact
- access more power from the lower body

- gain more awareness of the lower body, creating a more efficient kinematic sequence
- enhance internal and external hip rotation to reduce sway
- add rotation and control to your hip turn
- support full hip extension in your finish position

This following series of yoga poses will increase flexibility and strength in the hip flexors, internal and external rotators of the hips, gluteal muscles, quadriceps muscles, and hamstring muscles. Remember to integrate the core abdominal muscles before you begin any pose by drawing your navel toward your spine and lifting the ribcage up off of the waist. The focus of yoga is breathing, and proper breathing is the key to an effective flexibility program. Concentrate on deep diaphragmatic breathing in and out through your nose.

The Crescent Lunge Pose with the Golf Club

This pose strengthens the gluteal and quadriceps muscles and stretches the hip flexors, psoas muscles, and quadriceps muscles. It also stretches the feet and the Achilles tendon and improves balance.

- Hold a golf club in your right hand, resting the clubhead on the ground, and place your left hand on your left hip.
- Bend the right knee and place your right foot in front of you.
- Take the left foot behind you and lift high onto your left toes. Inhale as you slightly bend the left leg, engaging your left gluteal muscle, and press your left hip forward (see figure 8.11). Do not allow the

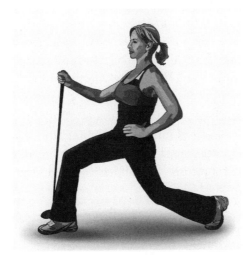

FIGURE 8.11

GUIDELINES FOR A SUCCESSFUL GOLF FITNESS PROGRAM

- *Be safe and start with a physical checkup.* Meet with your health care professional to see whether you need to consider any special modifications before starting an exercise program.
- *Work with a PGA professional.* If you are interested in improving your performance on the course, you need two coaches in your bag, a golf fitness professional who understands the mechanics of the golf swing, and a PGA pro who is willing to work with you on your game.
- *Set specific short-term and long-term goals.* Begin by meeting with your PGA professional to determine your golf goals. Have your PGA professional record a video or obtain 3-dimensional motion analysis of your swing. Perhaps you need more distance, better posture, or more core strength. Determine your short-term goals, like greater flexibility, more strength, or better balance. A long-term goal may be to alleviate a specific swing flaw.
- *Start slowly.* Rome wasn't built in a day. The good news is that the body responds very quickly to the slightest amount of flexibility conditioning.
- *Perform five to ten physical assessments.* This enables you to chart your success.
- *Do a little exercise multiple times a week.* Fifteen minutes of exercise four days a week will reap greater rewards than two hours on a Sunday. Be realistic about your time. Set yourself up for success.
- *Vary your workouts to keep you engaged.* Target specific parts of the body during each workout. Work your lower body and core and do cardio one day, focus on the upper body and core the next. Always warm up before your workout and prior to a round of golf.
- *Make a date, get a buddy, and create a support system.* Surround yourself with people who support you in your fitness program, and get a workout buddy. If you have an "appointment" to work out with a friend, you are more likely to show up and support each other in your goals.
- *Reward yourself.* Once you've reached your goal, treat yourself to something that reminds you of what a good job you've done and encourages you to continue. Make it something that supports your body, mind, and spirit, for example, a new driver or pair of golf shoes.
- *Seek support.* Use this book as a guide. Get a subscription to *Golf Fitness Magazine* and to golffitness-magazine.com for hundreds of tips on how to improve your golf game.

right leg to move beyond a 90-degree angle. Keep the knee directly over your ankle. Be sure to maintain an upright posture.

- For a more challenging pose, remove the club and place the hands on the waist. Inhale as you bring your right quad parallel to the floor. Exhale as you bring you right leg to the starting position.
- Repeat the move 10 times and switch legs.

The Adductor/Abductor "Window Washer" Stretch

- Lie on your back with your knees bent.
- Place your feet so that they are wider than your hips (see figure 8.12).
- Inhale as you lower your knees to the left (see figure 8.13).
- Exhale as you bring your legs back to the starting position.
- Repeat the move 10 times in each direction.

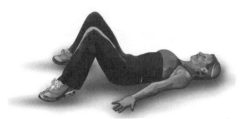

FIGURE 8.12

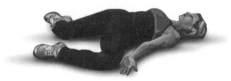

FIGURE 8.13

The Dynamic Pigeon Pose with a Stability Ball

- Place a stability ball at your feet and lie on your back.
- Lift your left leg and place your left heel on the ball.
- Bend the right knee and fold your right leg over and on top of your left leg, resting your right ankle on your left knee (see figure 8.14).
- Inhale as you pull the ball toward you, rolling it up your left heel (see figure 8.15). Focus on the stretch in the right gluteal muscle.

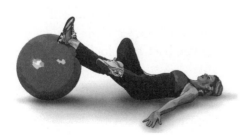

FIGURE 8.14

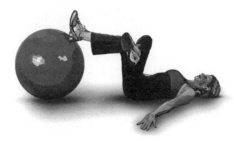

FIGURE 8.15

The complaint I hear from a lot of golfers is that their flexibility is gone and they feel like they don't make good turns. I tell people that they should combine flexibility with strength, and a great way to do that is power yoga and shaka yoga.

—JILL McGILL,
veteran LPGA Tour golfer

Be sure to keep your lower back on the floor. Try not to let the lower back arch.

- Hold for one breath.
- Repeat the move 10 times and switch legs.

The Importance of Recovery and Rest

Yoga can help your balance, an essential component in maximizing performance, whether you are on the golf course or in the boardroom. Many of us strive for more balance, both in our golf swing and our daily lives. In golf, when we are out of balance, it is glaringly apparent. We struggle, nothing seems to go our way, and as much as we try to shape our shots, it doesn't work, no matter how hard we try. When we are on the golf course, we instinctively know when we are in balance; our swing feels effortless, we hit the sweet spot perfectly, and the ball's trajectory is exactly how we imagined it.

In general, most golf fitness programs focus on building strength, endurance, speed, and flexibility—all key components to a comprehensive golf fitness program; however, we must devote part of our time to creating a balanced program, which includes recovery and rest. When we include recovery techniques, we reduce the physical and psychological stresses from golf and begin to maximize the full benefits of our workouts.

SUMMARY

Yoga and Pilates have numerous physical and mental benefits for golfers. Yoga teaches proper breathing and focus, that is, how to "be present" in your golf game. Pilates is an exercise system in which all work is based on the core, or center of the body, so all the muscles required for golf are trained during Pilates. Golfers who perform yoga and Pilates on a regular basis increase strength and stability and improve flexibility and balance (both mental and physical). These disciplines can also greatly improve your range of movement and power in your golf swing. Incorporating yoga and/or Pilates to your fitness routine can get you that smooth and powerful golf swing you have been looking for.

CHAPTER 9

NUTRITION FOR GOLF

Would you change the way you eat if you knew certain foods could help you play better golf? One area recreational golfers most often neglect is their nutritional intake before and especially during a round of golf. The saying the "wheels are falling off" usually comes midround, when you start to lose focus and your muscles start to fatigue. One way to alleviate this syndrome, so that you don't destroy an otherwise good round of golf or lose your shirt by pressing your skins partner when your energy levels are low, is to pay attention to what you eat and drink throughout the round.

Playing 18 holes can be downright draining, especially if you are in a competitive situation. Ask any Tour professional who makes a living playing golf, and they will tell you that tournament golf can be grueling and mind-numbing because of the need to maintain a high level of concentration and focus for four to five hours straight. After a few hours on the golf course, you may become fatigued and lose fine motor control over your body. Even a casual round of golf can be physically and mentally exhausting.

Managing your food intake and hydration levels and adding certain nutrients to your diet can not only help you concentrate and focus more on the golf course, it can also help you keep your heart rate steady as you make an important shot or putt, help your muscles fire faster for more power on a long drive, help you fight fatigue so you can play and practice longer, and even keep your blood pressure down to help you keep your cool after a bad shot.

GOLF NUTRITION 101: MAINTAINING YOUR ENERGY

The key to maintaining your energy level during a round of golf is controlling blood sugar. That means avoiding foods made with refined carbohydrates (white flour and/or sugars). Eating foods full of refined carbohydrates causes your blood sugar to spike sharply, so initially you feel alert and energetic. But after a while, your body adjusts, and your blood sugar drops, as does your energy. Suddenly, you don't feel as alert or as energetic as you did before. Instead, you feel tired, irritable, and confused. The refined carbohydrates are backfiring, causing your blood sugar to tank.

Eating the right preround meal levels off your blood sugar and boosts energy. Good foods contain no refined flour, sugar, or trans fats. Trans fats are found in foods made with hydrogenated oil and shortening, which are ingredients used in almost all baked goods and processed foods. Eating the right preround meal will help you play your best golf.

The following is an example of a healthy preround meal:

- 1 large apple, to provide the appropriate fuel for immediate energy.
- 3 eggs cooked in olive oil, to provide fat and protein for lasting energy.

The fat in the meal has the added benefit of slowing the emptying of the stomach, allowing the complex carbohydrates in the apple to be metered into the bloodstream more slowly.

We all know the importance of being fit, having proper swing mechanics, and using good equipment in having a good round of golf, but we sometimes forget the significance of eating the right foods so we can sustain our energy throughout the round to play our best golf. The best equipment in the world won't make a difference if you don't have the energy to get yourself around the course. We do not hear as much about nutrition for golf, but rest assured, the most elite golfers of the world follow specific diet regimens for the energy output they need to play their best.

This chapter is full of tips on nutrition, hydration, and energy management to help you sustain your highest energy level and play your best golf. We explain why a proper diet is so important in playing well for

18 holes and provide nutrition choices you can make at the course and a great snack recipe that you can make yourself to put in your golf bag.

FIVE NUTRIENTS THAT CAN HELP YOU PLAY BETTER GOLF

Not getting enough of certain vitamins and minerals can be a risk factor for chronic diseases and can impair your performance on the golf course. This section discusses some of the important nutrients that you should consider adding to your diet to help improve your game.

Calcium

- helps build and maintain strong bones
- helps muscles contract for a proper swing
- keeps the heart beating when anticipating an important shot or putt
- plays a role in nerve function

Where to Find It: milk, cheese, yogurt, calcium-fortified foods (bread, cereals, soy milk, and nutritional bars), tofu made with calcium sulfate, green leafy vegetables (kale, broccoli, and bokchoy)

Iron

- as part of hemoglobin, carries oxygen from your lungs to your cells
- keeps your immune system strong to help fight infections
- prevents anemia, a major cause of fatigue

Where to Find It: meats (liver, beef, chicken, and pork), fortified cereals and breads, pumpkin seeds, soybeans, spinach, legumes (kidney beans, black beans, pinto beans, lentil, and chickpeas)

Potassium

- helps fluid balance in the cells of the body
- assists in maintaining proper blood pressure to keep you cool under pressure
- aids in transmitting nerve signals
- helps muscles contract

Where to Find It: fruits (bananas, plums, peaches, apricots, oranges, and pears), potatoes, milk, legumes (kidney beans, black beans, pinto beans, lentil, and chickpeas), tomatoes, almonds, sports drinks

Omega-3 Fatty Acids

- reduces inflammation in sore muscles
- helps thin the blood and prevent clotting in and clogging of arteries
- aids in reducing blood pressure and triglyceride levels

Where to Find It: fatty fish (salmon, sardines, and herring), flax-seeds, canola oil, walnuts

B-Vitamins (Folic Acid, Thiamin, Niacin, Riboflavin, B6, B12, Pantothenic Acid)

- aids in producing energy in the cells of the body
- helps the body use sugars and fatty acids to enhance energy levels
- plays a vital role in making new cells for quick muscle recovery

Where to Find It: fortified breakfast cereals and other grain products, meats (liver, beef, chicken, and pork), eggs, vegetables, legumes (kidney beans, black beans, pinto beans, lentil, and chickpeas), milk

THE IMPORTANCE OF DRINKING ENOUGH WATER

Fatigue caused by dehydration can often result in a "blow up" on the back nine. Dehydration not only affects runners and professional athletes, it affects all of us in subtle ways, regardless of our physical condition. Being dehydrated is most noticeable on the golf course in the heat of the summer, but it can also sneak up on you on cooler days. Even though a cold beer sounds good during play, it can inhibit your concentration and dehydrate you. Even just one beer can impair your ability to focus and perform, especially on those all-important putts.

Effects of Dehydration

Golf is mainly a game of skill. If your focus and concentration are compromised, your game will suffer. We know that performance level decreases considerably if you are dehydrated. On a hot day, you are at a much higher risk of heat stress, which leads to heat exhaustion and heat stroke. Sweat losses of only 2 percent of your body weight can affect how your body regulates its temperature as well as your performance on the course. Weigh yourself before and after your round to see how much weight you lose.

Hot, dry weather can cause increased sweat loss, but humid weather can be just as dangerous because sweat does not evaporate from the skin, and you may not sweat as much as you think you do, since much of the moisture is coming from the air. It is best to get an early tee time in the heat of the summer.

Electrolytes

When you sweat, you lose water, but you also lose electrolytes, which include sodium, chloride, and potassium. These electrolytes are necessary for fluid balance, nerve impulses, and muscle contraction. You lose much more water through sweat than electrolytes; however, if you are sweating a lot, you should be sure to replace these electrolytes while you are on the course. Eating some fresh fruit, a sandwich, or a nutrition bar, or drinking a sports beverage a few hours into your round should do the trick of replenishing lost electrolytes.

How Much Should You Drink?

Fluid requirements vary from person to person and from day to day. Thirst is not a good indicator of when to drink. Instead, you should drink according to a schedule. It is best to drink 8 to 16 ounces 15 minutes prior to your round, 4 to 8 ounces every 15 to 30 minutes during your round, and 16 ounces following your round. If you have lost more than 1 pound during the round, you should drink an extra 16 ounces per pound lost.

ENERGY DRINKS: DO THEY REALLY DELIVER ENERGY?

Energy drinks are, in essence, soft drinks that either contain a form of sugar or artificial sweetener, caffeine, or various other ingredients. Energy drinks became a unique beverage category in 1997 when Red Bull was introduced into the United States from Austria. From 2001 to 2006, there was a 516 percent increase in the sale of energy drinks in the United States. The market hit $5.4 billion in 2007 and was expected to reach $10 billion by 2010. Sugar-free energy drinks have become one of the fastest growing segments of the energy drink market due to concerns of excessive caloric and carbohydrate intake from sugar.

The Anatomy of an Energy Drink

CAFFEINE

The main active ingredient in energy drinks is caffeine, a stimulant that activates the brain and central nervous system, giving us a burst of energy. Caffeine can come in a variety of forms, and many energy drinks contain guarana or yerba mate, which are both plants that contain caffeine.

Energy drinks are not as high in caffeine as you may think. Most have about 80 milligrams of caffeine in an 8-ounce can, and 16-ounce cans may have double that; however, some can have as much as 350 milligrams per can. To put this into perspective, the average cup of coffee has 140 milligrams per 8 ounces. A Starbucks tall, which is 12 ounces, contains approximately 250 milligrams of caffeine. A can of soda has between 35 and 55 milligrams of caffeine, while a cup of tea has about 50. The FDA does not require caffeine content to be printed on labels, so it is difficult to know exactly how much caffeine is in a beverage. Some energy drink websites reveal the amount of caffeine contained in their products.

Some studies have found that caffeine does indeed help improve cognitive and athletic performance, but most do not support a significant effect. The risks of excessive caffeine intake can outweigh the potential positive effects. Too much caffeine can cause high blood pressure, rapid heart rate, nervousness, irritability, sleeplessness, anxiety, and eventually ulcers. Most health organizations recommend a moderate caffeine intake of less than 300 milligrams per day, or about the equivalent of 24 ounces of energy drink.

SUGAR

Most energy drinks contain some form of sugar. Liquid sugar is the nutrient that gets into the bloodstream the quickest, offering instant energy. If you ever feel hypoglycemic (low blood sugar), you should drink juice or regular soda to get your sugar levels back to normal fast. But what goes up must come down, and when blood sugar rises quickly, it also falls quickly. "Energy drinks can give people a temporary buzz, but the effect is fleeting," said Dawn Jackson Blatner, a spokesperson for the American Dietetic Association and author of *The Flexitarian Diet,* during an interview. She continued, "But once the initial jolt wears off, people often feel more lethargic than before the drink." Some energy drink brands now offer sugar-free varieties. These do not contain sugar or calories but are made of artificial sweeteners.

B VITAMINS

To process energy in the body, certain B vitamins are necessary. Energy drinks add such B vitamins as niacin, pantothenic acid, pyridoxine, B12, and folic acid. While these vitamins are important for metabolism, increased amounts will not produce additional energy. If someone is deficient, the additional vitamins may help, but most people are not deficient, since these nutrients are abundant in our food supply and available in all multivitamins.

TAURINE

Taurine is a nonessential amino acid thought to improve reaction time and concentration. In most people, taurine is abundant in the body. Taurine is also found in meats and seafood.

GINSENG

Ginseng is an herbal supplement used to provide energy. Studies do not support the use of ginseng, and long-term side effects are unknown. Short-term side effects include inability to sleep, headaches, and increased blood pressure.

D-RIBOSE

Present in every cell in the body, D-Ribose is naturally occurring in the sugar needed to produce ATP, or energy in the body. Research is scant as to whether additional D-ribose in a supplement or beverage will produce additional feelings of energy.

L-CARNITINE

L-Carnitine is used by the body to break down fats to use for energy. Carnitine deficiencies are rare, and research has not revealed whether more is better.

The Potential Risks

Energy drinks are often heavily promoted to people involved in sports; however, they are not recommended to rehydrate after exercise due to their high caffeine content. Since concentration is such an important aspect of golf, a small amount of caffeine may enhance this ability during play; however, according to Blatner, "too much caffeine can negatively affect performance by making it difficult to focus and increasing nervousness and jitters."

If you have any medical conditions related to high blood pressure or heart disease, you should exercise caution before using any products that contain large amounts of caffeine or other stimulants. Caffeine has a half-life of six hours, meaning that only half of the amount of caffeine you drink is depleted after six hours. Since it can linger in your system for up to 12 hours after ingestion, you should not consume caffeine after noon, or it could affect your quality of sleep.

Energy drinks often contain ingredients that are not well studied in humans. For that reason, use caution with energy drink consumption. If you want to drink one, start out with a small amount to see how your body reacts. Everyone responds differently to food additives. The stimulating nature of many of the ingredients in energy drinks, especially when combined with alcohol, could have serious consequences.

The Bottom Line on Energy Drinks

Energy drinks may be harmless in small quantities for most healthy people; however, if you rely on these beverages to boost your energy, it is better to look into why you are feeling sluggish in the first place. Energy drinks are expensive and just don't live up to the claims their manufacturers make.

SNACKS THAT CAN IMPROVE YOUR GAME

Are you looking for the latest technology to boost your golf game? If so, look no further than your kitchen. Changing your eating habits before, during, and even after a round of golf may be just what you need to take your game to a new level.

Most golf lessons focus on teaching you the mechanics of the golf swing, which are certainly important, but to play your best, you should also focus on the mechanics of your body. This section details four healthy snack foods that can improve your overall well-being on and off of the golf course. Not only are they readily available and easy to prepare, they are easy to transport to the course. Keep these foods in your golf bag to help you play your best.

Eat Carrots to Improve Your Vision

Your vision is a key factor in playing your best golf. Eating carrots can enhance blood flow and function of the eyes. Improving your vision can help you gauge your distances, read putts, and see the ball in flight so that you can find it more easily.

Eat Tomatoes to Improve Your Endurance

Playing four or five hours of golf requires a tremendous amount of endurance. Since tomatoes are loaded with lycopene (an antioxidant the body uses to dispose of toxins, fight disease, and repair tissue), eating tomatoes before you play golf can help improve blood flow to the heart and increase your endurance so that you can play your best the entire round.

Eat Walnuts to Improve Your Focus

Walnuts are one of the best plant sources of protein. They are rich in fiber, B vitamins, magnesium, and antioxidants like vitamin E. Nuts are also high in plant sterols and fat, most importantly monounsaturated and polyunsaturated fats (omega 3 fatty acids, the good fats), which have been shown to lower LDL, or bad cholesterol, levels. Eating walnuts while you play can help improve brain function and focus.

Eat Celery for Stronger Bones

Strong bones are essential for having a strong body. Increasing your strength will not only help prevent injuries on the golf course, but it will also help you hit the ball farther. Celery contains a large amount of sodium, which helps feed bones to make them stronger. If you are sodium deficient, your body will pull its reserves from your bones, making them brittle. Keep your bones strong and your swing powerful by eating a few celery sticks during your round.

VITAMINS AND SUPPLEMENTS FOR GOLFERS

Can we as golfers improve our performance by adding nutritional supplements to our daily routine? The answer is yes. GFM contributors Diego Gorosteroga and Brad Brewer share what research has proven to be the best supplements to help increase strength, prolong endurance, improve mental focus, and reduce inflammation in joints and supporting tissue.

For the past decade, nutritionists have warned of free radicals in our drinking water, air, and food, thus the need for nutritional supplements to fuel and cleanse our bodies is greater than ever. Food alone cannot deliver sufficient nutrition to live a healthy and active lifestyle. Such nutrients as protein and minerals are the essential building blocks for strong tissue, injury repair, flexibility, and strength. Stamina and the ability to focus depend on well-balanced levels of blood sugar and fluids. When your blood sugar and electrolyte levels drop, so does your ability to concentrate. No matter how good your technique, you will begin to make errant shots costly to your final score.

To improve your health and ability to perform, the following are some over-the-counter supplements that can aid in your quest for consistent high performance both on and off of the golf course:

1. *For strength:* Tyrosine is an amino acid that can be used to effectively maintain the neurotransmitters in the brain for heavy resistance activity. Protein supplements come from a variety of sources that we will address separately. Whey protein is an easily digestible protein. It has a higher insulin content and works best when taken after a round of golf to replenish reserves used during the round. Casein and egg protein work well when ingested during the round to maintain steady insulin levels. Those who are lactose intolerant should go for the egg protein, as it is also the easiest to digest and the most bioavailable for our bodies.

2. *For endurance:* Complex carbohydrates supply the energy needed for endurance. Foods that have a low glycemic index prevent insulin spikes and drops that can cause jitters and low energy.

3. *For mental focus:* Tyrosine, whey protein, casein, egg protein, and complex carbohydrates can also help you maintain focus during your round due to the fact that brain function largely depends on glucose and insulin levels in the body. The level of focus we are trying to maintain determines how much glucose is supplied to the brain. Ginko biloba has also been proven to increase the ability to maintain focus. As a long-term supplement for improved focus, fish oil can improve mental clarity and overall function.

4. *To fight inflammation:* Fish oil and proceolytic enzyme can consume the debris from trauma to tissue and improve the rate of recovery. Arnica Gel is a great topical supplement for bruises and soreness after a round of golf or a heavy workout. The newest "super food" from the Amazon jungle is the Acai Berry, which is found in such products as Monavie, a potent antioxidant.

Supplements alone cannot meet the complex requirements of the human body; however, optimum nutrition can be achieved by combining a variety of vegetables, fruits, whole grains, lean protein, and low-fat dairy products with supplements taken according to their recommended dosages.

WHAT'S IN YOUR SNACK BAG?

Maintaining your energy during a round of golf is crucial in playing your best. A sharp drop in energy makes you feel tired, listless, and confused, and can you cost strokes and turn a good round into a bad one. Eating the right snacks during a round can work wonders. In addition to being good for you, healthy snacks can boost your energy level and increase your concentration. The following is a list of six good snacks for golfers:

1. peanuts or seeds
2. beef jerky
3. string cheese
4. apples
5. home-popped popcorn
6. low-carbohydrate nutrition bars

Planning ahead also helps maintain blood sugar. Eat a balanced portion of protein and fat before playing. Add some carbohydrates in the form of whole foods (whole grains, vegetables, or fruit), and you're good to go. This combination of foods stabilizes your blood sugar and energy levels.

BANANAS: THE PERFECT
SNACK FOOD

If you are serious about shaving strokes off your score, it is important to pay attention to the kinds of snack foods you put into your mouth on the golf course. Snacks high in fat and sugar can zap your energy and affect your concentration. Instead of grabbing a bag of chips or a candy bar at the halfway house, stock your golf bag with bananas.

Bananas are considered by many to be the perfect snack food. Bananas contain three natural sugars, sucrose, fructose, and glucose, combined with fiber. A banana provides an instant, sustained, and substantial boost in energy. Research shows that just two bananas can provide enough energy for a strenuous 90-minute workout or four-hour round of golf. It is no wonder that the banana is the number one fruit for some of the world's leading athletes.

The benefits of bananas include the following:

- Bananas contain tryptophan, a type of protein that the body can easily convert into serotonin, which helps you relax, improves your mood, and generally makes you feel happier. Eating bananas can help you shrug off those occasional bad shots.
- Bananas contain vitamin B and vitamin B6, which help regulate blood glucose levels and calm the nervous system. Healthy glucose levels and a calm demeanor can help you keep your energy levels up while you play and keep you relaxed so you can play your best golf.
- Bananas contain loads of the vital mineral potassium, which helps keep your muscles hydrated and you alert on the golf course.
- Bananas are high in fiber and have a natural antacid effect on the body, which helps restore normal bowel action and keep nervous stomachs in check.
- Bananas are known to have anti-inflammatory properties. Try rubbing the inside of the banana peel on an insect bite to reduce swelling and irritation.
- Bananas are convenient and easy to store in your golf bag, and they come complete with their own biodegradable wrappers.

Throw a couple of bananas in your golf bag the next time you play.

FOODS TO HELP YOU FOCUS ON THE GOLF COURSE

If you have trouble concentrating on the golf course or lose all focus and miss what should be easy shots, it could have something to do with what you are eating and drinking before and during your game. If you want to be able to concentrate better on your swing, start to focus on the food going into your body, and you will see improvement in your game. Eating something before you tee off is vital to your focus throughout the game.

Carbohydrates are your brain's preferred fuel source, so it is best to eat something that contains carbs at least an hour or two before you tee off. It is also a good idea to mix in a bit of protein and fat. You should try to eat something every three or four hours, so if you ate breakfast an hour or two prior to your tee time, you should have a snack during play. Pack something healthy so you don't have to rely on the snack cart and the potential nutritional disasters waiting there for you.

Getting the Proper Nutrients

Studies show that certain nutrients foster increased memory, focus, and concentration. This section explores foods that contain the nutrients most beneficial for the game of golf.

B Vitamins

B vitamins help your body produce energy within its trillions of cells. They include niacin, thiamin, riboflavin, folate, B6, and B12. In recent studies, folic acid has been shown to improve cognitive function, and it may help prevent Alzheimer's disease. B vitamins are found in grain products (bread, cereal, and pasta), wheat germ, legumes (kidney beans, black beans, pinto beans, lentil, and chickpeas), nuts, seeds, eggs, dairy products, lean meats, poultry, fish, and a variety of fruits and vegetables. This nutrient is abundant in our food supply.

ANTIOXIDANTS AND PHYTOCHEMICALS

These naturally occurring plant substances help keep your brain sharp and may preserve brain cells. They help kill off free radicals that attack your cells, helping to maintain healthy brain cells. Antioxidants and phytochemicals are found in fruits (especially in berries, apples, oranges, grapefruit, lemons, cherries, and melons), vegetables (especially spinach, broccoli, peppers, onions, asparagus, potatoes, and sweet potatoes), legumes (kidney beans, black beans, pinto beans, lentil, and chickpeas), whole grains, and nuts and seeds.

OMEGA-3 FATTY ACIDS

These "healthy fats" are good for brain development and function. The DHA in omega-3s is found in the brain, and studies show that omega-3s may actually help build the brain's gray matter. These acids are found in fatty fish (especially salmon, sardines, herring, mackerel, and tuna), ground flaxseeds, walnuts, fortified eggs, and other fortified foods.

CHOLINE

Choline is an essential nutrient that we hear little about. It has been shown to help with memory and in maintaining and building healthy brain cells. Choline is found in egg yolks, peanuts and peanut butter, lettuce, cauliflower, and soy lecithin.

Meal and Snack Ideas

The following are some healthy meal and snack ideas for before or during your game. These foods are high in carbohydrates but also have some protein and fat and contain at least one of the nutrients listed above.

MEALS

- whole-grain toast with an egg or peanut butter and a piece of fruit
- one half of a whole-grain bagel with light cream cheese, smoked salmon, and a slice of tomato and onion
- smoothie made with milk (or soy milk), fresh berries, one tablespoon of soy lecithin granules, and one tablespoon of ground flaxseed
- cottage cheese and fresh fruit
- whole-grain cereal, milk, and a banana or berries
- oatmeal made with milk and fresh berries
- veggie omelet with whole-wheat toast
- turkey sandwich on whole-wheat toast with lettuce, tomato, and fruit salad
- chef's salad with low-calorie dressing and a whole-wheat roll

WHEN AND WHAT TO EAT BEFORE YOUR NEXT ROUND

Golf is played at all times of the day, so you may not have time to sit down for a traditional breakfast if your tee time is at 7 a.m. or get lunch before your noon tee off. Some avid golfers would rather skip a meal than miss their round of golf, but missing meals means that many players end up running on empty on the course or stuffing their faces after the round at the 19th hole, neither of which is a good idea. So what should you eat before a round of golf?

When you start a round of golf, you should feel neither starved nor stuffed. You don't want to eat immediately before you tee off or practice, because it may lead to cramping and bloating. It is hard to make a complete turn if your stomach is full. Conversely, playing golf on an empty stomach may cause you to run out of energy by the time you make the turn.

Your best bet is to eat a light snack or meal about one or two hours before your round. Choose something high in carbohydrates and protein and lower in fat. Some examples of good preround fuel include a bagel with peanut butter; a banana and an energy bar, a bowl of cold cereal with a cup of milk, or a small turkey sandwich. Stay away from such rich, fatty, or high-sugar foods as hot dogs, hamburgers, french fries, potato chips, and candy bars.

Try to eat a light snack every few hours during your round, and be sure to stay hydrated, drinking small amounts of water every few holes. Take the time to fuel up before and during your next round. It may help you play your best golf ever.

SNACKS

- one banana
- one apple
- handful of grapes
- one nutrition bar
- half of a peanut butter and jelly sandwich
- one cup of trail mix (dried fruit and nuts)
- one fruit leather
- one granola bar

Go Nuts On and Off of the Course

Besides being convenient and tasty, nuts and seeds have a variety of health benefits. Many people avoid nuts because of the high fat and caloric content, but there are numerous other beneficial components of nuts that make eating them worthwhile.

Golfers are unique athletes because of the low intensity but long duration of the sport. "Nuts are beneficial for golfers as a snack to maintain energy levels and keep them satisfied throughout their game," stated Amy Jamieson-Petonic, a spokesperson for the American Dietetic Association and sports nutrition specialist, during an interview. Nuts are convenient and easy to pack in the golf bag and won't spoil in the heat. Because nuts can give you long-lasting energy, they can keep you mentally sharp, something very important when you are trying to make those tough putts.

The following are a few nut facts:

- Walnuts are the richest known food source of melatonin, a hormone with powerful antioxidant properties to fight disease.
- Peanuts are actually not nuts, but rather a legume, and they grow underground, unlike nuts, which grow on trees.
- A total of 80 percent of the world's pecans come from the United States, with Georgia leading in their production.
- Almonds cannot grow unless their blossoms are pollinated by bees, so almond growers bring in beehives during blooming season.
- To get the omega-3 acid from inside a tiny flaxseed, you need to grind it or chew it well.

COMPONENTS OF NUTS AND SEEDS

The Food and Drug Administration approved a health claim stating that, "Scientific evidence suggests but does not prove that eating an ounce and a half per day of most nuts, as part of a diet low in saturated fat and cholesterol, may reduce the risk of heart disease."[1] The type of fat found in nuts is unsaturated, either in the form of monounsaturated or polyunsaturated fat. Walnuts and flaxseeds are particularly high in alpha linolenic acid, a type of omega-3 polyunsaturated fat found to reduce blood pressure and inflammation and prevent plaque buildup in arteries. This is good news for heart disease prevention, but also for the golfer looking for a natural anti-inflammatory. "Research has shown promise in using omega-3s to reduce inflammation in people with arthritis, a big concern for golfers," said Jamieson-Petonic. Nuts and seeds also contain plant sterols, which research shows helps to reduce LDL, or bad cholesterol, levels.

Calories

Although nuts and seeds are high in calories, they do not seem to lead to weight gain. Studies on walnuts, almonds, and peanuts have shown that people can substitute nuts for other fats in the diet with positive results. When nuts are added, the subjects studied reported feeling more satisfied, helping them to control the total number of calories they were eating that day. The fiber, protein, and fat in nuts all contribute to feelings of satiety, or fullness.

Fiber

Nuts are a tasty and convenient way to boost your fiber intake. They contain soluble fiber, but mostly insoluble fiber. "Insoluble fiber is great for promoting digestion, while the soluble fiber acts like a sponge soaking up cholesterol," said David Grotto, author of *101 Foods That Could Save Your Life*, during an interview. Grotto also pointed out that the fiber in nuts aids in blood sugar control.

Nutrients

Nuts are high in selenium and vitamin E, both of which act as antioxidants, protecting our cells from damage. Most nuts also contain some magnesium, copper, and vitamin B6. All nuts have some phytonutrients, but each type of nut is slightly different in the nutrients it contains. For that reason, it is a good idea to eat a variety of nuts.

JUST A HANDFUL A DAY

Because nuts taste so good, it is easy to go overboard with portion size. Just a small handful, or about an ounce, is the correct serving size for most people. The number of nuts that fits into an ounce varies per nut. "A handful of nuts every day may keep the doctor away, the scale at bay, and you golfing another day," said Grotto.

The following are a few creative ways to add nuts to your day:

- Spice up your oatmeal with some chopped walnuts, pecans, or almonds.
- Make any salad more exciting with added whole or candied nuts.
- Add ground flaxseed to smoothies, muffins, and quick breads.
- Throw some chopped walnuts into your blueberry pancakes.

NICK FALDO'S PREROUND AND POSTROUND FUEL

Still athletically competitive, 2008 Ryder Cup captain and seven-time major championship winner Nick Faldo plays a limited schedule between his many endeavors, so when he does play, he wants to perform his best. Faldo works out regularly and knows the importance of good nutrition to build proper muscle function and help his endurance and stamina for golf. As with his practice and on-course strategy, Faldo is meticulous about his diet. He knows that golf requires a substantial amount of energy, so he loads himself up with the correct amount of carbohydrates, protein, and healthy fats before and after he plays.

Faldo's Preround Fuel
- muesli and a banana
- porridge and honey
- toast (whole meal bread)
- bagels with bananas
- pancakes (whole meal flour)

Faldo's Preround Snacks (2 Hours Prior to Tee Time)
- raisin muffins
- rice cakes
- bagels
- whole meal bread

Faldo's Preround Snacks (30 Minutes Prior to Tee Time)
- bananas
- cup of raisins
- malt biscuits
- jelly beans
- energy bars
- carbohydrate drinks

Faldo's Postround Snacks (5 to 30 Minutes Following a Round)
- carbohydrate drinks
- energy or fruit bars
- bananas
- jelly beans

Faldo's Preround Meal for an Afternoon Tee Time (2 Hours Prior to Teeing Off) or Postround Meal (2 Hours Following a Round)
- rice
- potatoes
- baked beans
- noodles or pasta

- bread (whole meal, pita, bagels)
- fish (tuna or salmon)
- chicken
- hummus
- peanut butter
- ice cream
- yogurt

- Instead of peanut butter, try Sunbutter (sunflower seed), almond butter, soy nut butter, or cashew butter.
- Top your low-fat frozen yogurt with chopped pecans or peanuts.
- Make your own granola using flaxseeds, almonds, pecans, and oats.
- Mix various nuts with dried cherries, blueberries, and cranberries.
- Grind pecans and mix them with bread crumbs to coat fish or chicken.
- Toss pine nuts (or any nut) into your favorite pasta or rice dish.

EASE INFLAMMATION WITH THE RIGHT FOODS

Have you ever had a sore shoulder after an intense round of golf, or a "bum knee" that requires repeated doses of anti-inflammatory medication? New research on inflammation reveals a link between painful joints and muscles and such chronic ailments as heart disease, cancer, and a depressed immune system. The studies also offer significant promise of relief for those suffering from inflammatory conditions. Reduced inflammation can mean reduced pain, which is welcome news for anyone suffering from a painful condition.

Inflammation 101

Inflammation is an internal reaction to injury or infection. Tissue in the body becomes inflamed in a healing effort to stop the spread of injury or infection. Inflammation can happen anywhere in the body. Sometimes you can see and feel inflammation, while other times you cannot. For instance, you can see a cut get red or an ankle swell after a sprain, but you cannot see your internal organs when they become inflamed. You cannot feel the vessels in your heart, but they can also become inflamed. Some common conditions associated with inflammation include irritable bowel syndrome, pneumonia, arthritis, gout, cancer, fibromyalgia, and such allergies as hay fever.

Researchers believe that eating certain foods may contribute to inflammation, while other foods may reduce it. Diet alone may not replace the use of anti-inflammatory medications or treatments, but including foods that can decrease an inflammatory response can certainly help reduce recurring inflammation, especially that which leads to chronic disease.

Foods That Can Cause Inflammation

Foods that are thought to cause inflammation are those high in unhealthy fats and simple sugars and low in nutritional value. They include the following:

- *Saturated fats:* Foods high in saturated fat include such dairy foods as cream, ice cream, and cheese; fatty cuts of red meat; coconut oil; and palm kernel oil. Certain fatty acids, like arachidonic acid, present in saturated fats promote inflammation. These acids also stick to arteries, leading to plaque buildup.
- *Trans fats:* Foods high in trans fats include hydrogenated oils found in deep fried foods like crackers, donuts, and cookies. These synthetic fats lead to atherosclerosis, or the thickening and inflammation of the arteries.
- *Sugar:* Sugar is found in such foods as sweetened beverages, desserts, and candy. A diet high in sugar can cause a spike in blood sugar and a surge of insulin, causing an inflammatory response in the body.
- *Refined grains:* White bread, white rice, and white pasta are all made from refined grains. These grains have been stripped of much of their nutritional value and fiber, causing a similar blood sugar/insulin response as sugars.
- *Nitrites:* Processed meats like deli meats, hot dogs, and sausages contain nitrites. These chemicals can cause cell damage and lead to inflammation.
- *Alcohol:* Alcohol can be found in beer, wine, and liquor. While small amounts (one drink per day) may have potential health benefits, larger amounts can contribute to inflammation. Even two drinks per day has been linked to higher levels of inflammation and certain disease risks.

Anti-inflammatory Foods

- *Omega-3 fatty acids:* Salmon, trout, herring, tuna, certain eggs, flaxseeds, walnuts, and canola oil all contain omega-3 fatty acids. Research strongly suggests that omega-3 fats are anti-inflammatory powerhouses.
- *Monounsaturated fats:* Monounsaturated fats can be found in olives, olive oil, canola oil, nuts, and avocados. These healthy fats should replace saturated and trans fats to reduce inflammation.
- *Antioxidants:* Berries, grapes, cherries, apples, pears, beans, artichokes, potatoes, cabbage, peppers, spinach, tomatoes, and broccoli all contain antioxidants. Tea, coffee, whole grains, nuts, and spices are also good sources. Antioxidants help to kill off free radicals, which cause inflammation and damage cells.
- *Whole grains:* Whole-wheat bread, quinoa, brown rice, millet, oats, barley, corn, and rye are all made from whole grains. These grains are also high in antioxidants, and the fiber in them helps reduce inflammation.
- *Lean protein:* Lean protein can be found in skinless white meat poultry, lean beef, lean pork, low-fat dairy, eggs, beans, and soy. Since protein helps build and repair tissue, it is essential in injury repair and the reduction of inflammation.

Tips for Maintaining an Anti-inflammatory Diet

1. *Aim for five to nine servings of fruits and vegetables daily.* One serving is one half cup cooked or one cup raw. Try to get two servings at each meal and additional servings at snack time.

2. *Choose whole grains over refined grains.* At least three of your daily servings of grain should be whole grain.

3. *Aim for two to three servings of low- or reduced-fat dairy per day.* Choose low-fat yogurt, skim or 1 percent milk, or reduced fat cheese.

4. *Get one or more servings of beans each day.* Beans are high in soluble fiber, and red beans contain the most antioxidants of all the vegetables. Choose from kidney beans, red beans, pinto beans, black beans, garbanzo beans, cannellini beans, great northern beans, lima beans, black-eyed peas, and lentils.

5. *Eat fish.* Aim for a serving of fatty fish at least three times per week. A daily serving is even better. You can get omega-3s from flaxseeds, walnuts, and canola oil, but fish is the richest source of EPA/DHA, the healthiest kinds of omega-3s.

The following is a sample diet plan for a day on the course:

Breakfast
- oatmeal with ground flaxseed
- blueberries
- skim milk
- cup of tea or coffee

On the Golf Course
- bananas
- water

Lunch
- mixed greens salad with red peppers, sun-dried tomatoes, artichokes, olives, garbanzo beans, feta cheese, and balsamic vinaigrette
- black bean soup
- whole-grain roll

Snack
- reduced-fat string cheese
- whole-grain crackers

Dinner
- roasted potatoes tossed with olive oil, rosemary, basil, and oregano
- sautéed spinach and garlic with golden raisins
- grilled salmon with lemon
- baked apple with cinnamon

Supplements

While getting nutrients from whole foods is always better than getting them from a pill, since you are getting the synergistic effect of all of the health-promoting components of the food, it isn't always possible to get all the necessary nutrients you need in one day. In addition, if you are not a fish eater, taking a supplement containing omega-3 fatty acids in the form of fish oil has been shown to be beneficial. Taking 1,000 to 2,000 milligrams per day of omega-3 fatty acids in the form of DHA and EPA has proven to be most effective; however, you should not exceed 3,000 milligrams per day, as higher levels may increase the risk of hemorrhagic stroke. If you are taking other medications, you should check with your doctor before you start a regimen of omega-3 supplements.

IS THE 19TH HOLE
RUINING YOUR GAME?

Everyone looks forward to the famous 19th hole. Even if you shot poorly in the previous 18 holes, the 19th hole is one that not many people miss. But loading up on the wrong foods will not only prevent you from recovering properly, it could ultimately affect your waistline and health.

Although you are expending lots of energy on the golf course, it doesn't take much food or drink to put those calories right back into your body. Eating a healthy snack and drinking plenty of water or other sports beverages while you are on the course will keep you hydrated and fueled.

After a round of golf, you should be hungry, thirsty, and ready to eat a solid meal. The best way to recover is to eat a nutrient-rich mix of foods within an hour after finishing. The following are some important components of postgame fuel:

1. *Hydration.* Even if you drank while on the course, it is likely you are still slightly dehydrated from being out the sun, sweating, and physically exerting yourself. Alcohol and caffeine act as diuretics (dehydrators), so neither is a good choice after a round of golf. The best choice is water; however, since iced tea and soft drinks contain little caffeine, you could also choose one of those beverages, in addition to a glass of water. Just be aware of calories if you choose sweet tea or regular soda. If you have a beer, mixed drink, or glass of wine, order a tall glass of water to go along with it for hydration.

2. *Antioxidants.* Although you used sunscreen (right?), the sun can still have damaging effects on your skin. Sun exposure causes your body to create large quantities of free radicals. Heavy exercise and pollution also have the same effect. The best defense against these free radicals are antioxidants. Load up on fresh fruits like berries, apples, and plums and such vegetables as artichokes, beans, broccoli, spinach, and potatoes. And don't forget your whole grains and nuts, like pecans or walnuts.

3. *Carbohydrates.* You just worked really hard out on the course and expended a lot of energy. Your body's preferred source of energy is the carbohydrate, and the energy you have stored for short-term use is glycogen. While on the course for many hours, you dipped into that glycogen, and now that you are finished you need to replenish it. Eat plenty of complex carbohydrates, like bread, potatoes, rice, beans, or pasta, within an hour after you finish to replenish lost glycogen.

4. *Protein.* Protein is vital in building and repairing the muscles you used during your game. Protein is rich in amino acids, which replenish muscles to prevent injury. Consume protein-rich

foods, which include beef, poultry, pork, eggs, cheese, milk, soy, and beans, to get your muscles ready for the next round.

5. *Omega-3 fatty acids*. Many golfers suffer from various levels of inflammation, and foods rich in omega-3 fatty acids can help reduce this inflammation. These foods include such fatty fish as salmon, sardines, rainbow trout, herring, flounder, and tuna. You can also get omega-3s from flaxseeds, walnuts, and canola oil, but they are not as powerful as the fish-based omega-3s. If you don't like fish, get a fish oil-based omega-3 supplement.

The following are a few examples of good 19th-Hole Meals:

Postround Snack
- 8 ounces of yogurt (for protein and complex carbohydrates)
- 2 tablespoons of chopped walnuts (for antioxidants, omega-3s, and protein)
- 1 cup of fresh berries (for antioxidants, complex carbohydrates, and hydration)
- 16 ounces of unsweetened tea (for hydration and antioxidants)

Postround Lunch
- 2 cups of spinach or other salad greens, with artichokes, tomatoes, and peppers (for antioxidants)
- 5 ounces of grilled salmon (for omega-3s and protein)
- 2 tablespoons of light Italian dressing
- 1 whole-wheat roll (for complex carbohydrates)
- 16 ounces of water (for hydration)
- 5 ounces of red wine spritzer (for antioxidants)

Postround Dinner
- 4 ounces of lean roast beef (for protein)
- 1 whole-wheat pita (for complex carbohydrates and antioxidants)
- spinach, tomatoes, and shredded carrots in a sandwich (for antioxidants)
- mustard and 1 tablespoon of canola oil mayonnaise (for omega-3s)
- 1 fruit cup (for antioxidants, carbohydrates, and hydration)
- 16 ounces of diet soft drink or sparkling water (for hydration)

Supplements containing antioxidants have not yet been proven effective. Phytochemicals are naturally occurring plant substances that also have antioxidant-like effects on your body. Eating fruits, vegetables, and whole grains is the only way to ensure you are getting the recommended amount of antioxidants and phytochemicals.

SUMMARY

Why worry about what you eat before, during, and after your round of golf? Because what you eat can determine whether you play a mediocre round of golf or a great round of golf. In this chapter, we presented numerous examples of preround and postround meals to help you optimize your nutrition to help you play your best golf. Your nutrition determines your endurance and stamina, which are crucial in helping you play with consistency and power throughout the round.

CHAPTER 10

THE MENTAL GAME

Golf fitness is important in helping you achieve more power, improve your swing mechanics, prevent injury, and extend your playing career. But to play your best golf and shoot your lowest scores, you also need to work out your mind. It is important to give the same attention to your inner body as your outer body. When you start a golf fitness program, you should begin by assessing your body's strengths and weaknesses. The same goes for starting a mental golf fitness program. You should begin by assessing your mental game's strengths and weaknesses to figure out which areas you should concentrate on. Do you have an overactive mind that thinks negatively rather than positively? Do you spend more time analyzing and tinkering with your golf swing while you play than assessing the shot at hand? A mental golf assessment can help you determine your on-course playing temperament, your on-course strategy and management style, as well as your mental strengths and weaknesses. Learning more about your playing style can help you build a golf mental system that can pinpoint the areas you need to improve.

For years, professional golfers have been working with sports psychologists to improve their mental games. Tour professionals know the importance of positive self-talk, visualization, relaxation techniques, and developing a rock solid preshot routine. Even professionals have trouble controlling their nerves, and they look for ways to help them perform at their best.

This chapter contains tips and techniques to help you play your best under pressure, learn to focus and relax on the golf course, learn to set goals, develop a preshot routine, adopt easy practice methods, conquer your first-tee jitters, trust your swing, and play your best golf and have fun doing it.

YOUR FIRST SHOT: MAKE IT YOUR BEST

In his classic book, *Golf My Way* (1974), the great Jack Nicklaus states that the opening tee shot is perhaps the most critical shot in golf.[1] The Golden Bear goes on to say that he always takes a little extra time on the first tee to create a mindset that ensures that he is going to make his first shot his best. He sees his first shot as the kingpin of the beginning of a great day, and he likes to do everything he can to get off to a confident start.

GFM contributor and sports psychologist Dr. Robert K Winters, affectionately known as Dr. Bob, specializes in sports and personal performance training and has extensive training in sports psychology, motor and visual learning, sports vision, sports medicine, and educational psychology. Winters couldn't agree more with Nicklaus. "Nothing is more satisfying than stepping onto the first tee and hitting the ball where you want it to go. After you hit your opening tee shot and it sails down the middle of the fairway, it tends to stabilize you mentally and emotionally for the following shots and builds confidence for the entire day," says Winters.

Not only does a square hit provide immediate positive feedback about your swing mechanics, it also reinforces a feeling of being in control. Hitting your opening shot squarely accentuates a strong sense of swing competence and helps you gain trust in your swing; however, for many golfers, the ability to get off to a solid start from the first tee is difficult.

Which category do you fall into? To find out, ask yourself the following questions:

1. Are you a fast or slow starter? Do you always seem to hit the first shot well?
2. Does it take some time for you to get your game and composure under control?
3. Do you need to play two or three holes to feel at ease?
4. Do you find it hard to step up onto the first tee and feel comfortable while others are watching you?

If you often get off to a great start, good for you! However, if you are a slow starter and feel uncomfortable on the first tee box, the number one culprit is probably nervous tension and anxiety. This feeling is increased by the thought of having others watch you perform. Being under the watchful eyes of others creates a form of social evaluation that most people are not comfortable with, similar to the anxiety and fear involved with public speaking.

Another reason for poor first shot performance is the expectation of a new round and the hope and value we place on the result before we even hit the first ball. Having high expectations of what could be is a large threat to just enjoying your round and focusing on your task, which is to hit your ball solidly and play golf.

The next section details strategies for preparing your mind and body to be more confident and get off to a solid start. The strategies include the following:

1. Warming Up
2. Letting Go of Others
3. Taking Control of the Tee Box
4. Making a Rehearsal Swing
5. Allowing Yourself to Trust
6. Accepting the Result

Strategy 1: Warming Up

One of the best ways to develop a feeling of being "ready" when you step up to the first tee is to get yourself sufficiently warmed up by hitting a few balls during your warm-up session. Hitting a number of successful and solid shots on the warm-up range creates a feeling of positive readiness. It is amazing to see the number of players who step onto the first tee and expect to hit a great shot without warming up, something that is unheard-of in top amateur and professional tournaments. Touring professionals usually take 30 to 45 minutes to warm up their minds and bodies before they walk to the first tee and would never think about starting a round before being adequately stretched and warmed up. Neither should you. Always take the time to warm up properly.

After you have warmed up and worked your way to hitting the driver, take 10 balls and imagine playing through the first three holes of the course during this warm-up session. Start with a driver, then perhaps hit a 7-iron, and follow it up with a chip. Then hit a 3-wood or 4-iron (depending on whether the hole is a par 3, 4, or 5). Continue until you have played the first three holes. Using this strategy, you can walk onto the first tee having already "played" the first three holes and just continue your round.

Strategy 2: Letting Go of Others

Does having an audience on the first tee make you anxious because you think they are watching you? Perhaps you are overly concerned with what they might be thinking, or you want to impress them and show them how far you can hit the ball. Or, you may just want to get off the tee without embarrassing yourself and ruining your reputation as a pretty good player. Do these scenarios sound familiar?

When a player steps onto the first tee and is overly concerned with what others are thinking, he or she is immersed in the "evaluation syndrome." This syndrome is an affliction of misdirected focus and attention. Rather than being focused on the task of hitting the ball to the target, the golfer is intimidated by what others may or may not be thinking. This leads to self-directed thoughts, which in turn leads to "trying to impress." When a golfer is trying to impress others or becomes worried about what others may say or think about his or her performance, the golfer becomes detached from the target, and the swing is affected. Rather than a swing that is fluid, the swing becomes forced and effortful. The result is ineffective motion and poor timing. The player is lucky if he or she even hits the ball. All of this is caused by placing too much thought and energy into what others think about you and your golf game.

The remedy for this syndrome is relatively simple. You must detach yourself from everyone around you the moment you step onto the tee. You must understand that no one else really cares what you do (or don't do) on the tee box. Many people think that once they're on the tee, all eyes are on them, but most players are really just disinterested bystanders waiting for you to hit the ball so that they can stand up and begin their 30-second tee-off ritual. It is important not to take yourself too seriously and put yourself into a paranoid mental state. Rather, get yourself focused, go through your preshot routine, and take care of your business, which is to hit the ball down the middle of the fairway to your target.

Strategy 3: Taking Control of the Tee Box

Consistent with strategy 2, this strategy suggests that when you step onto the first tee area, you should remind yourself that this is your area and that you will allow nothing to interfere with you, your thoughts, or your swing. Recognize that once you step onto the tee box, it is a "safe area." This "safe area" mentality permits you to focus on your target (the fairway) and not allow your thoughts and eyes to drift back into the crowd mingling about on the first tee. This strategy will help keep you focused on the upcoming shot and not worry about what others may be doing or saying.

Take your time, and be a bit more deliberate when it is your turn to hit the ball. Rushing around and hurrying to "get it over with" only raises your tension level on the first tee. Take a couple of deep breaths, tee the ball, and go into your preshot routine. By doing so, you are consciously and subconsciously allowing your body to calm down, which also helps clear your mind for the upcoming shot.

Strategy 4: Making a Rehearsal Swing

One of the most consistent findings in the sport science literature is that preshot routines help prepare the body for physical movement. They also help to focus the mind, body, and eyes on the target, for a more automatic performance. With this in mind, make a rehearsal swing during your preshot routine that simulates the same motor action for the real performance. This rehearsal swing helps "preset" a sequence of motion that helps "grease the wheel" for the actual swing.

Oftentimes, when you go to the first tee without a warm-up or rehearsal swing, you are swinging "cold" and may be at risk for pulling or straining your muscles. The effectiveness of the swing can also be limited, because no prestretched reflex movement has been created. Also, by using an active rehearsal swing, you can monitor the pace of your movement and fine-tune your thoughts. Part of being on automatic pilot is not thinking about the movement process. By preprogramming the right movement in your active rehearsal swing, all that is left to do is step up and replay that same motion without conscious effort or thought. Thus, the actual swing is merely a reflexive effort, versus one that is forced or manipulated.

Strategy 5: Allowing Yourself to Trust

Allowing yourself to trust in golf means trusting your mechanics when it is time to swing. An idea that has been used throughout the years (especially by Jack Nicklaus and other great stars) is to use a swing key or simple thought that helps focus your attention on one particular aspect of the swinging motion. It doesn't matter what you use, just keep it simple and consistent. Using too many swing keys only distorts the process and confuses your brain. In golf, the simpler you can keep the thought process, the more consistency and success you will achieve.

It is also helpful to take a couple of cleansing breaths and move the shoulder and neck muscles as you inhale and exhale. The next time you see Fred Couples play, notice how he always hikes up his shirt and sleeves and loosens his neck and shoulder muscles. This allows him to take a deep breath and make that wonderful and flowing shoulder turn characteristic of his golf swing. Don't feel that breathing control is too New Age, because research suggests that muscles that are soft and freshly oxygenated move easier and with less resistance than those that are constricted and haven't been freshly oxygenated. Remember, if Tiger Woods is doing deep breathing before big tee shots, you should too.

Strategy 6: Accepting the Result

Finally, understand that whatever the outcome of the opening tee shot, it is yours for that day and that round. Acceptance is the final component of every good routine. Until you can accept and move on, you cannot have closure on the shot. Too many players carry their anger from the opening shot over to subsequent shots, until they have done irreparable harm to their psyche and their scorecards. You must learn to accept your results (good or bad) and move on to your next shot with renewed vigor, and do so quickly. Accepting "what is" and moving onto the next shot is vital in staying in the present moment and playing your best golf.

Veteran PGA Tour player Allen Miller once stated that when you are on the first tee, "Do not allow yourself to be influenced by others, or what I liken to be known as 'the committee of them.' The only person who can make a difference in your game today on the course is you." Know that you have a confidence-building strategy. This strategy proposes that you step up onto the first tee in control. It also suggests that you do not have to worry about what anyone else is doing or thinking. Simply tee your ball and make a good swing and know that you have executed your first shot with confidence and a sense of purpose.

SEVEN MENTAL MISTAKES ALL GOLFERS MAKE AND HOW TO OVERCOME THEM

You keep thinking the same thoughts, you keep getting the same results, and somehow you're still wondering why things don't change. Owner of Golf Mind Power and GFM contributor Randy Friedman thinks you should keep reading. According to Friedman, your thoughts produce the shots you hit, and your shots give you the feelings you feel,

THINK YOURSELF AROUND YOUR HOME GOLF COURSE

George Bernard Shaw once said, "People hate thinking. They will do almost anything to avoid it. I have made an international reputation for myself by doing it once or twice a week." In the age of sound bites, instant messages, and text messaging, contemplation is becoming a lost art. "People want quick tips to fix their swings. Many say that they don't even want to have to think on the golf course, so they end up playing mindless golf, repeating the same mistakes round after round," says Karen Palacios-Jansen, GFM contributor and LPGA teaching professional.

Do you mindlessly play your home course, not thinking or planning each shot? Do you automatically assume that you know the correct yardage when you arrive to your ball? Do you tee off the first hole without a plan or goal in mind for your round? When was the last time you mapped out the perfect strategy to play your home course? Do you carry notes in your bag about each hole? To break out of your rut and improve your handicap at your home course, you need to think yourself around the course. Before your next round, spend a few moments contemplating your strategy and planning your round of golf. You spend a lot of time and money on the golf course, so isn't it worth it to make a plan for yourself?

The following are a few pointers for contemplating before your next round:

- *Set a goal for the round*. Your goal could be to break 90 or 80, to hit as many fairways and greens as possible, to take no more than two putts on every hole, to have fun, and so forth.
- *Decide where to aim and land your tee shots on each hole*. Mapping out each hole is a good way for you to practice your game without even going to the golf course.
- *Decide where to lay up on par 5s and par 4s*. Wouldn't you rather lay up to the 100-yard marker and have a full swing into a green rather than have to make a 40- or 30-yard half pitch shot?
- *Make a list of positive swing thoughts to refer to throughout the round*. It is okay to have swing thoughts. Jotting down a list of tips will help remind you of what things you should be working on in your swing.
- *Study the greens, and jot down fall lines and severe breaks*. Spend some time mapping out the greens on your home course so you don't have to guess which way a putt will break.

Having a thoughtful plan of how to play your home course can be your key to shaving shots off of your next round of golf.

good and bad. He says that if you keep thinking what you're thinking, you'll keep getting what you're getting. To play better golf, you must think better thoughts. Professionals in any sport know how to perform under a range of pressures. In this section, Friedman gives us seven common mental mistakes (that golf professionals rarely make) and tells us how we can learn to think more effectively to improve our game.

1. "Just Think Target . . . and Finish the Swing . . . and Pause at the Top . . . and Hold the Angle . . . and Keep My Eye on the Ball . . . Oh, and Don't Sway"

How many times have you hit balls at the range before your round, found your groove, and decided on a swing thought for the day, only to change it on the first tee? Or better yet, how many times have you used that swing thought on the first tee, hit one poor shot, and then changed your swing thought? Here commitment is the key.

Failing to commit to a single mindset is one of the most common mistakes Friedman sees with students of all levels. It is very important to be consistent with your swing thought. Once you have a routine and a game plan, be brave and stick with it, no matter what. The more you change your thoughts, the more your thoughts change your swing, and the more variance in the shots that come off the clubface. When you commit to a positive thought, you detach yourself from fear and move into a place of fun, love, and joy.

2. "I Don't Like This Club, but I'll Hit It Anyway!"

While holding a club, have you ever found yourself thinking, "I don't like this club, but I'll hit it anyway!"? Do you think professional golfers think that way? Probably not. Most pros have an internal light bulb that tells them right away that the club they are holding doesn't feel right. If you have ever watched golf on television and seen a Tour player going back and forth with the caddy figuring out which club to hit, it's because they are looking for the feeling that says, "yes, this is the one." Then, and only then, will they hit the shot without trepidation. Doubt creates fear, and fear does not make for a good golf shot.

Your mental and physical games must be in agreement before you can hit your best shot. If your external "you" (the physical) doesn't agree with the internal "you" (the mental), *you* will cancel each other out and have no shot. We all have an internal light bulb within us, and that is your awareness. Once you become aware, you are halfway there. The next time you play, make an effort to be more aware. Notice what you are feeling as you take your club out of the bag. Your goal is to feel good before you hit the shot. This "yes" will put you in agreement with your inner mental swing and your outer physical swing.

3. "I Can't Play Well When I'm Nervous"

Tiger Woods has said that if he wasn't nervous on the first tee, he'd be nervous. The difference is that his nervousness is a positive energy feeling that he uses to get his round started. Most amateurs think that being nervous is a bad thing. They connect negative energy to this nervousness and hope the worst won't happen.

The reality is that you can play great golf and give brilliant business presentations when you are nervous. The real enemy is negative thinking, combined with nervousness. You can regain your power by breathing deeply and attaching feelings of love before you play. Think about the beauty of the golf course, the nature surrounding you, and the appreciation of where you are at that moment. When you attach the word *love* to your game, your negative feelings will disappear and be replaced with positive ones. Before your next round of golf, say, "I love playing golf, I appreciate everything about the golf course, and I look forward to every shot I hit." Your nerves will thank you.

4. "I Hope I Don't Hit It in the Water Again!"

Professionals rarely make the same mistake twice. Granted, they may (and should) take more calculated risks than a recreational golfer, but if something is not working that day, they usually won't repeat it. How about you? Do you learn from your mistakes and make better choices the next time around? One of the biggest mental mistakes amateur golfers make is coming up short of the green.

The next time you play, take more than enough club to get over a hazard. It's better to be on the back of the green (having taken more than enough club), than to be short in the water or bunker. When you've gone over the green a few times, then dial it down a club.

5. "I Can't Figure Out These Greens. These Greens Are Too Slow . . . These Greens Are Too Fast . . . These Greens Are Just Right!"

Can you guess what the professionals think about as they examine the greens during their round of golf? What about you? How do you consider the greens as you evaluate your putting results? If you think about it, what options do you really have? You have no choice but to accept the greens as they are.

You can either accept the condition of the greens on the course you are playing on that day or beat yourself up and never figure out the speed of the greens. The sooner you accept the speed of the greens, rather than wish you could change them, the sooner you will putt well on them. The next time you are on the practice putting green, say to yourself, "I love these greens, they are perfect for me." Then take that thought with you to the golf course.

6. "I Just Can't See the Shot!"

Most low-handicap golfers imagine their shot in their mind before they actually hit it. And although all of us have the ability to imagine, we don't always tap into it. We are all born with the gift of imagination, but not many people use it past their toddler years. If you haven't reaped the benefits of using imagery in golf, you're not tapping into your true potential.

Seeing yourself perform in your mind can help prepare you for actual play. Imagery can work with little practice. The more you practice visualizing, the better you will be at it. Just as hitting balls at the driving range is your physical practice, visualizing your shot before you hit it is your mental practice. As you fall asleep tonight, play 9 holes in your mind. See every shot you hit with detail. Watch patiently as the ball climbs into the sky, from each tee box to each green, until you pull the ball out of the last hole. Practice helps performance.

7. "I Hate Playing with This Person, They're So . . ."

Can you imagine if Tiger, Ernie, or Phil complained about being paired with someone they didn't like and moaned about it during the entire round? As comical as that sounds, many golfers complain (out loud, as well as quietly to themselves) about who they have been paired up with. This creates a negative feeling from the first tee that can easily ruin your entire round. Has this ever happened to you?

Acceptance is a powerful tool that can neutralize negative emotions. It's up to you to accept your partner, whether it is for fun or competition. A great way to stay focused and play your game is to decide on a goal you want to accomplish for that day. For example, you can keep stats of how many fairways and greens you have hit, track how many putts you have had on each hole, or strive to shoot below a certain score for 9 or 18 holes.

By doing this, you limit your distractions and focus more on your game. Appreciating the beautiful nature surrounding you and your love of the best game in the world is another great way to keep you happy playing your game. Incorporate these seven mental tips into your game, and watch the magic unfold.

WINNING: IT'S A MATTER OF BALANCE

Every golfer wants to win, but do you play golf to win for the sake of winning, or are you more interested in developing your talent? According to Bob Winters, if you play for recognition and personal glory, you probably have a strong ego orientation for golfing achievement. You may play to be the top-ranked player at your club and are revered as the "player to beat." Winters says that the excitement and recognition that you derive from your athletic success on the golf course may elicit a sense of increased self-worth and high golf self-esteem. If you view golf in this way, then golf is the vehicle for delivering your wants and desires into feelings of personal success and self-validation.

On the other hand, if you are more concerned about self-improvement and want to achieve a higher level of ball striking and game consistency, you are exhibiting traits of a mastery orientation for golf achievement.

Players who are mastery-oriented play golf for the satisfaction of getting better and are willing to put their egos aside while improving their baseline levels of competence. Many golf instructors prefer working with mastery-oriented golfers and consider them to be serious students of the game, because they are motivated to practice their basic motor skills and patient enough to realize that it will take time to develop competency in terms of measurable performance. Many golfers with a strong ego orientation just don't want to wait for success, abandon the improvement process, and feel that if something is not broken, why fix it?

In addition, a golfer who has a mastery orientation is not out to merely beat the competition, rather they are there to hone their ball striking skills so that they can face the challenge of golf, beat the golf course, and defeat "Old Man Par." By improving their skill competency, they are able to hit more consistent shots and lower their scores so that they can enjoy the game even more.

A Balanced Approach

So, what should you do? Do you have to make a choice between the differing orientations based on your personality or golfing goals? For instance, is it entirely bad to have an ego orientation? Is it okay to want to improve your game and at the same time want to win and be a great competitor? Do great golfers have a combination of both orientations? These questions abound much like the old philosophical question, "Which comes first, the chicken or the egg?"

In this framework and different from the old fable, neither ego orientation nor mastery orientation comes first or second. Neither is better or more favorable than the other. The orientations and styles that people adopt are as different as the people who play golf. Individual differences and perceptual biases play more important roles than simply knowing one's overall game orientation. It is how one interprets and perceives their objectives that helps make a golfer a player of the game versus one who merely uses golf as a recreational device.

The basic truth is that both ego and mastery orientations are components of high-level achievers in golf, but obtaining a healthy balance between the two is vital for long-term success, both on and off the golf course. If you are a tough-minded competitor, you need to have the consummate golf skills required to put you into the hunt consistently, and you need for those skills to hold up under pressure. That means you are always looking and striving to create an edge in your golfing performance. In this sense, you are always looking for ways to improve your baseline golf motor skills, while at the same time maintaining your current level of golf performance.

If you are looking to develop your talent to your utmost potential, a good way to measure your progress is to continually place yourself in achievement situations where your performance can be evaluated and scored. Therefore, both ego and mastery orientations contribute to your overall development as a ball striker and a complete player of the game. You can probably find as many golfers who are ego driven and have an absolute thirst for wanting to improve their motor skills so they can be more effective in competition as there are mastery-oriented golfers who want to strike the ball more consistently so that they can enjoy competition even more; however, there is one golfer who blends the two approaches into a balanced and formidable approach, and that is Tiger Woods.

TIGER WOODS: A BALANCE OF EGO AND MASTERY

Tiger Woods is the poster boy for a balanced approach to a winning golf mindset. Tiger is the perfect blend of the tenacious competitor who is always hungry for another win and the golfing student who is always trying to improve. From the time he was a young golfer under the watchful eye of his father, Tiger has played in every event with the idea that he was the golfer who was going to play to win. Even in his early PGA career when asked what he wanted to do on the PGA Tour, his answer was simply to win. And winning is what Tiger Woods does best. Tiger plays to win and does the best he can in everything he enters. When Tiger is in the field, many (if not most) of the competitors view him as the man to beat. Tiger's playing philosophy of "I play to win, and I refuse to lose" has served him well for more than two decades of competitive golf at every level.

But the roots of success and golf orientation go deeper than that. Even when Tiger is off the golf course and relaxing at home, he is competitive in everything that he does, whether it is playing basketball, ping pong, or even video games. The simple truth is that Tiger plays to win because for him, winning is fun. Winning on Tiger's terms is the thrill of pushing himself to the edge of competitive fire (even when he suffers severe pain and injury), because at the end of the day, he knows he did what he set out to do, and that is to be the ultimate athletic warrior who is still standing and leading after everyone else has putted out and gone home.

However, even with Tiger's extreme competitive fire and egotistic nature, we must also understand that he is a serious student of the game who is always looking to improve himself in any way he can. Tiger's evaluation of his play and progress is not about comparing himself to other players, it is about Tiger measuring himself against his own potential for greatness. Woods has repeatedly told the golfing world that he is always looking for and finding new ways to make himself better and that the day he stops learning how to improve his performance is the day he will leave the game.

This attitude is reflected in his ability to make swing changes that take weeks, months, and even years to bear fruit, while at the same time pushing himself in the weight room to improve his physical fitness and stamina. Tiger is a wonderful blend of a balanced approach of ego and mastery orientations. This has allowed him to become the ultimate golf performer.

So what are some ways that you can create a feeling of improvement, while at the same time creating an atmosphere for success in evaluative situations and golf tournaments? The following section offers a few thoughts to help you win more consistently and create a feeling of confidence on the course, whether you are playing for fun or are in the middle of a competition.

SEVEN KEYS FOR DEVELOPING A WINNING MINDSET

Whether you have an ego or mastery orientation, the bottom line is that everyone wants to win and feel good about their golf game. The following are seven strategies you can implement to create a winning mindset that balances both the ego and mastery orientations of playing golf:

1. *Make a grade report for each club in your bag.* Give yourself a letter grade that corresponds with your consistency, square contact, and accuracy with that club. If you have any club or shot in your bag with a score of C or worse, you should spend time working with that club or on that shot to improve your competency. Make a list of other areas of your game that need some work, for example, bunker play, trouble shots, and wedge shots around the green. If any of these areas get a grade of C or worse, you will know what you need to work on.

2. *Plan your course strategy the night before the tournament, and go through each hole shot by shot.* By charting out a course the night before a tournament and becoming familiar with the particular demands of a hole, you can create a mental edge for the next day because you have

prepared yourself with a specific shot strategy. This preplanned strategy will allow you to become more confident and composed when you actually face that particular hole. Being mentally prepared makes you ready to swing for your target with trust, because you have already created a mental blueprint for success.

3. *Practice specific shots that you will need on the course that you are about to play to eliminate inconsistency and build confidence.* By examining the demands of the course and the setup, you can take the appropriate steps to develop the competence to master the shots that will most likely be required during your round. By practicing specific shots that you are likely to have to execute, you will have a sense of readiness and not be caught off guard with an unexpected shot situation.

4. *Remind yourself that the upcoming round is about your performance and golfing enjoyment.* It is not about trying to play perfect golf, impress your playing partners, or beat the top-ranked contenders. The idea is to be fully engaged in every shot you make. When you enter the clubhouse gates, smile and remind yourself that today you are going to be the most upbeat and emotionally stable golfer on the course. Having an optimistic perspective is a good way to get your day off to a great start.

5. *Commit yourself to the moment.* It is psychologically and physiologically imperative that you commit yourself to each shot with full intention and purposefulness. Become clear about what you want to accomplish. Committing to your decision about how to play a shot before you step into the ball will help create feelings of confidence and control.

6. *Take the time to assess and evaluate what it is that you want to accomplish.* One of the most common mental mistakes that golfers make is that they rush their process and do not take enough time to thoroughly analyze the situation. They inevitably make an unforced error in physical execution. It is important to remember that in any preshot routine, the most important component is that you get to a *yes* mindset and completely trust that the ball is going to your intended target.

7. *Accept your result after you hit your shot, no matter what the result.* It is crucial to remember that once a shot is hit, it is over. That shot is history. It is finished. It is up to you to accept the result and move on. Focus your energy on the next shot and how you can improve your performance moving forward.

Developing a winning mindset is about finding a workable balance between your ego and mastery orientations for playing top-level golf.

Make it a priority to make your day on the course a day of passion and the pursuit of achieving excellence, instead of trying to beat others or being perfect. Do not allow yourself to be distracted by the games of score or by comparing yourself to other competitors. Rather, commit yourself to becoming engaged with your target and accepting of your mistakes. Enjoy your good shots and move on. You will find that having a balanced mind and attitude will lead to more winning days on the links.

BUILDING POSITIVE MOMENTUM FOR GREAT GOLF

In such sports as basketball and football, when a team is on a "roll," they generally talk about "momentum" being in their favor. Athletes have spoken of this psychological effect for years. When they feel the emotional and physical flow changing in the game, they talk about how they have "changed jerseys" and how they are now the ones ready to deliver an offensive blow to their opponent. This effect can be seen in basketball, when a player gets a "hot hand" and makes shots from anywhere on the court, and in football, when the team with the positive "MO" moves the ball at will when they are on offense or stops the other team from advancing when they are on defense.

This same feeling is also found in golf. Every golfer, at one time or another, has experienced positive momentum, regardless of talent, handicap, or playing ability. Positive "MO" is an exhilarating feeling of confidence that comes with a series of successful shots or putts during the round. It is a feeling of power and intensity, yet it is associated with an accompanying sense of calm and self-control. When the world's number one player, Tiger Woods, is "on a roll," he can both sense and feel it, but almost every golfer and fan who is watching him is also captivated by the raw emotion of this positive athletic force.

Many of the world's most elite players will tell you that when they experience positive momentum, they feel completely in control, like they can make the golf ball do whatever they want. They speak about having a feeling of omnipotent control and how easy the game becomes, almost as if they can do no wrong. It is little wonder then that Tiger, Phil, and the rest of the top touring professionals in the world do everything they can to extend this feeling of positive momentum. You can tap into this feeling as well.

On the other hand, golfers can also experience negative momentum. We have all felt the effects of negative "MO" during a round of golf, which is generally characterized by the sick feeling you get when you miss a series of short putts or after a few of your shots go haywire. This feeling often serves as a confirmation that your game is slipping away and that your confidence is fading as well.

As we are playing, we often ask ourselves how we can stop this mental and emotional bleeding. The truth about momentum is twofold, containing both bad and good news. The bad news is that as a golfer, you're going to miss drives, iron shots, and putts. This is almost a certainty. The reality of playing this wonderful game is that you will make mistakes and that you will have to face the challenge of not folding your emotional tent when things start to go poorly. Many players talk about becoming frustrated and discouraged when they miss an important putt or hit a poor shot. We are all vulnerable to the forces of negative momentum on the golf course.

The good news is that you can learn to stop negative momentum, turn the negative thoughts and feelings into positive ones, and build a foundation for creating positive momentum and lower scores. The following are two important tips to help you turn negative MO into positive MO:

1. *View your game as being on a continuum.* Understand that positive momentum can quickly morph into negative momentum, or somewhere in between. It is your job to keep your emotions and momentum going in a positive direction with positive thoughts, behaviors, and attitude. When things are going well, trust that good things will continue to happen and keep swinging for your target. Remind yourself that you deserve success. Visualize yourself being successful, and imagine that all

of your drives and shots are going to the pin and that all of your putts are going to fall in the hole.

As PGA and LPGA Tour players say, "Keep striking while the iron is hot." Don't stop to analyze how well you're doing, keep going forward. Don't look around and compare yourself to your competitors or playing companions or stop to check your scorecard. Stay in the now, and keep playing the way that you have been playing.

As surfers have long known, "if the wave swells, ride it all the way to the shore." The same is true of positive momentum in golf. Don't allow yourself to sit back and dwell on the good feelings after a series of good shots. It is not the time to become mentally lazy and satisfied. There will be more than enough time to reflect on the good aspects long after the round is over.

2. *Be patient.* If you feel that nothing good is happening in your golf round and that you are just going through the motions, hang in there, play within yourself, and keep telling yourself that the momentum is about to shift. Ancient Eastern philosophy suggests that we do not create an event to happen, but that the event happens because we have waited for the opportunity to arise. You must do the same. This is a long-term approach to your golf game.

By staying focused in the present, making clear and committed decisions about the shot at hand, not forcing things to happen, and playing within yourself, you allow the moment (or momentum) to build, thus when the moment presents itself, by virtue of staying positive and patient, you will have created a new "wave" to ride, and the movement of positive golf momentum starts once again.

Building positive momentum is similar to the surfer who rides an ocean wave. He rides it as long as the swell takes him forward, and when the swell or wave dies, he waits for the next "swell" to come along, and he gets up and rides again. If the surfer falls or crashes into the ocean or shoreline, he just gets up and starts the process all over again. The same can be true of your golf game. When you are doing well, keep playing until the bubble bursts. On the next shot (after a missed shot or putt), start fresh, knowing that with this new shot, a purposeful and direct movement toward building success has started once again. Creating positive psychological momentum is a never-ending process and one that allows you to play your most consistent and lowest-scoring golf ever.

Building and sustaining positive golf momentum is a continual process of understanding your game and allowing yourself to play the way you know you can play. Being aware of your momentum will help you be patient and allow you to build confidence. Because golf is played over the course of several hours, there are many opportunities (and much time) to go hot and cold. The greatest tournament golfers in the world know the value of building positive momentum right from the start and trying to sustain and build upon those positive feelings over a period of four or five hours. They also know the value of turning their thoughts and feelings from a negative into a positive mindset. Remember, creating a positive mindset is imperative in preventing you from falling prey to negative thoughts and feelings, and, more importantly, in creating positive psychological momentum. May you always focus your energy on playing with positive golf momentum.

USING YOUR MIND TO MAKE GREAT PUTTS

We all know the cliché, "You drive for show and putt for dough." The truth of the matter is that great players know that if they make putts, they will be in the hunt to win championships, but if they putt poorly or have an average day on the greens, their chances for success are greatly diminished. This is why one of the most important things you can have when you step onto the first tee is the internal feeling that you will putt well the entire day. Knowing that you have the proper "touch and feel" helps create a foundation for success that carries into all aspects of your game. In fact, knowing that you are prepared to play and putt well is one of the most important assets in building your confidence level.

As LPGA player Vicki Goetze-Ackerman once said, "If I practice and warm up the right way, then I normally feel prepared and have confidence." Goetze-Ackerman says that her physical, mental, and emotional preparation allows her to perform with confidence. She builds her confidence by planning her practice and warm-up time so that she can accomplish specific goals of feeling good about her ball striking and putting. By doing so, she creates a climate of positive feelings and thoughts by virtue of her warm-up and preparation.

While Goetze-Ackerman takes time to create positive feelings for herself, most golfers fail to plan for their success. According to our own Dr. Winters, a great number of amateur golfers do not take the time to consider that they have the ability to prepare themselves for success.

With that in mind, Dr. Winters would like for you to take a bit of time and reflect on your golfing past and your best putting round. Try to remember when you had a "hot" putter or when you were seeing your ball roll gently into the cup. Did you believe that you could make every putt? Did you concentrate well? Did you feel in control? What started the belief that you could make every shot that day? Did you have a nice flow during your preputting routine? If you can tap into your memory bank and retrieve these thoughts and emotions, you may find yourself able to rekindle wonderful feelings that can work their way back into your golf psyche the next time you take your putter out of your golf bag.

Positive Reminders for Success

Reminding yourself that you have the capability to think good thoughts and make good decisions about the line and speed of a ball is a good place to start if you have had putting problems in the past. Taking the time to reflect on your past and draw on good memories helps create a positive mindset and reemphasize good feelings with the putter.

If you do not have any good memories of putting success, it is important that you think about the things that you can do well. For example, are you good at getting a good read of the putting surface and looking for contours and tilt? Are you savvy at making a clear decision of the ball-roll line? Do you excel at knowing how hard you need to hit the ball to get it to roll on your ball-roll line? Are you good at contacting the ball squarely and having a smooth, accelerating stroke? Are you proficient at adhering to your putting plan and routine? The point is that you have to start somewhere to create these positive feelings of confidence, and there is no better time to start than right now.

The Mind of a Great Putter

Dr. Winters says that one of the most important pieces of information from his research in putting psychology during the past 25 years is crystal clear: Great putters think, believe, and create their own good thoughts about great putting. Great putters are always talking and thinking about making putts and putting great, even if they are missing, because they realize that missing is a part of putting. The flip side of the coin is that poor putters think, believe, and create negative thoughts about their putting. Poor putters are always talking, complaining, and thinking about how bad their putting is. In such cases as this, the dominant thought one holds in the mind becomes reality.

It is no secret that the main difference between great putters and poor putters is their perceptions of self-thought, self-talk, and self-image. One group views themselves as successful, while the other group views themselves as failures, thus what you think about most comes true. Therefore, you have a choice: You can think about changing yourself into a great putter and create good thoughts and feelings for success, or you can think that you are doomed to putt poorly for all eternity and feel sorry for yourself and putt indifferently at best. The choice is yours.

It was for this very reason that the late legendary golf teacher Harvey Penick told his two star pupils, Ben Crenshaw and Tom Kite, to go out to dinner with good putters and players. The reason was simple psychology. The good putters were always talking about making putts, while the poor putters were constantly complaining about the greens and making excuses for their inability to drop the ball into the hole. Just by "hanging out" with the good putters, Crenshaw and Kite gave themselves a chance at successful input just by being exposed to the positive thought processes of others. Penick knew the value of a positive and directed mind long before golf psychology a career field.

The following are a few tips from Dr. Winters on how to warm up your mind for success that will help build a foundation for your putting confidence.

Imagine Success on the Green

Perhaps the best place to create positive thoughts and feelings is in your bed just before you fall asleep. As the saying goes, "A picture is worth a thousand words." In the case of getting yourself ready for a great putting round, let's say, "A picture is worth a thousand putts!"

One strategy is to imagine that you are putting great and playing with a lot of putting confidence. As you lie in bed the night before a big match or tournament, take a couple of deep breaths and clear your mind of the days' activities. Remain motionless for a few minutes, and focus on the pattern of your breathing. Visualize yourself at the golf course as you walk onto the first green and with feelings of confidence. View yourself as a player who looks as if he or she knows that the putts are going to fall into the hole. Imagine going through your preputting routine and seeing yourself setting up and addressing the ball with the sole purpose that the putt is going down.

Continue to see yourself performing confidently as you take your last look at the hole and bring your head and eyes back to the ball. Finally, see yourself making a smooth stroke as you hit the ball squarely and solidly. Watch the ball roll down the line with the proper speed, and see it fall into the cup. Relive this picture over and over again. Build a foundation for success by seeing yourself as always being successful in your mind's eye. This allows you to see that picture again the following day on the green. You can preprogram yourself for putting success via your imagination, thus you can create your own blueprint for success simply by thinking good thoughts about your putting. Everyone who has ever been successful on the golf course or won their first tournament had to picture themselves as a winner in their mind first. The actual performance followed the thought.

Become a Positive Putter

It seems like a cliché to remind yourself to stay positive, but the truth of the matter is, if you can't be enthusiastic about your own success, no one else is going to be excited for you. It is important to understand that there is real power in positive thinking, and there is even greater power in the world of negative thinking. What we know from sport psychology literature is that you can be positive and try hard and still not be successful; however, the real power of negative thinking is that if you believe in negative thoughts and feelings, it almost always works.

Using positive thinking and maintaining a positive attitude gives you the opportunity to see how great a putter you can be. If you use the negative approach, you won't even make it onto the first green before your golf day is over. Your putting success is reliant on your ability to stay enthusiastic, upbeat, and positive. Never criticize yourself or be judgmental of your putting prowess.

Remind yourself as you drive through the front gates to your club or golf course that you are going to believe in your putting ability and become your best buddy on the green, versus doubting yourself and being your worst enemy. This strategy alone will help your putting success immeasurably. It is also helpful to remind yourself to be patient and composed, even when the putts don't drop.

LPGA Tour star and 2007 European Solheim Cup captain Helen Alfredsson once said, "I know that I am going to miss putts, but I am going to miss them while trying to make them." This attitude has given Alfredsson the knowledge that her mind is focused on making putts and that she can accept whatever happens. The game of golf doesn't have to become a *you* versus *you* situation. It can be a game of *you* for *you*. Become your best partner, ally, and coach on the golf course, because doing so allows you to create an attitude for success and maintain your playing focus and composure.

Warm Up Your "Mental Oil"

Many golfers don't take the time to warm up on the putting green or get a feel for the speed of the greens. You might see them go to the practice green, take three balls, drop them down, and start putting to a hole 20 feet away. They putt the first ball, and it slides by on the low side about 15 inches to the left of the hole. The second and third balls aren't much better, and the result is that this player has just hit three putts and experienced three misses. This is not a good way to develop feel and touch for the upcoming round, and it certainly doesn't provide a foundation for building putting confidence.

The following system was developed by Dr. Winters to help get the "mental oil" flowing for a round:

1. *Start by rolling some long putts approximately 30 to 40 feet toward the far part of the green (no target focus, no putting cup).* Just hit the ball solidly, and watch it roll over the green. Warming up with a few long putts to no specific target allows you to work the "kinks" out of your system and concentrate on making solid contact with the ball without judgment or critical thinking. This procedure is similar to the one carried out by race car drivers who drive around the track at speeds of 50 to 70 miles an hour prior to a race. They are simply getting their car's oil warmed up for the big performance, when they will be racing around the track at 250 miles per hour or more.

2. *After hitting five or six long putts back and forth without judgment or target focus, hit a few 20- to 30-foot putts to the edge of the putting green for distance and speed control.* If you can successfully place six balls within one foot of each other in a tight dispersion pattern, you can feel confident that you have fine-tuned your distance control.

3. *Move to a putting cup or hole, place 3 balls 12 inches away from the hole, and stroke the 3 balls into the hole.* This is an important step, because your first mental pictures for the day are of making a putt. You can see, hear, and feel the golf balls going into the cup, and you are starting the day off on a positive note.

4. *Next putt with just one ball, and use your preputting routine to try and hole some 10- to 15-foot putts.* Putting one ball from different distances will help you get into "playing mode" and improve your focus, green reading, and decision-making capabilities for the round. Complete 8 to 10 trials at this 10- to 15-foot range As PGA Tour player Bob Estes once said, "You are going to get more out of your

practice and warm-up if you make it more like what it is going to be on the course."

5. *Once you have completed your 10- to 15-foot range trials, hit some longer putts at different lengths (20, 30, or 40 feet) to evaluate your distance control.* Remember that the warm-up is the place to fine-tune your mind for making putts, but it is not the competition. Tune your touch and feel, and do not allow yourself to become distracted with mechanical thoughts. Focus on the ball rolling into the putting cup.

6. *After you are satisfied with your distance control, make three 3-foot putts in a row before you proceed to the first tee.* Holing three short putts and seeing the ball go into the hole helps give you a positive image in your mind of your putting competence when you walk to the first tee.

When walking onto the first green, remind yourself that you have prepared yourself mentally, emotionally, and physically to putt well and that you are ready to do some great putting. Don't place huge expectations on yourself and think that today is the day that you start to putt great or else. Rather, on each and every putt, know that your mind is giving your body the proper thoughts and signals to respond appropriately and that this is giving you the greatest chance to be successful on the green.

One of the key elements of a great putter is the feeling that he or she has earned the right to be confident. Preparing yourself mentally, emotionally, and physically helps instill feelings of competence and thoughts of success. Give yourself a chance to see how great a putter you can be by looking inside yourself and understanding that great putting is more a matter of personal choice of attitude than just mechanical stroke aptitude. Throughout the history of the game, the greatest putters have known the importance of practicing their mechanics and fine-tuning their touch and feel, but they also never forgot to warm up their mental oil and attitude for a great day of putting.

SUMMARY

Mastering the mental side of the game of golf is one of the key elements for playing better golf and enjoying your time on the golf course. Making small changes in your way of thinking can make a dramatic difference in your score. Managing your thoughts, being patient, and having clear mental goals will greatly improve your chances of scoring your best. Managing your mental game, along with your physical game, will give you the edge to play your best golf.

CHAPTER 11

THE HEALTHY GOLFER

The Advisory Team at GFM is not only dedicated to sharing the best and latest information on improving your golf game, we are also committed to helping you improve your health and well-being. Leading a healthy lifestyle is not only good for you, but it will also contribute to a better golf game. Any time you improve your health and well-being, you increase your chances of playing better, because your body moves better so you can swing more efficiently and focus and concentrate more on the golf course. Your mood and disposition also improve so that you can relax and enjoy yourself more.

Our goal is to help golfers lead healthy lives so that they are able to prolong their golf careers, play golf more often, and compete without pain. Maintaining a healthy weight, getting enough sleep, and keeping our minds as fit as our bodies are the keys to playing our best each time we tee it up, and improving our quality of life. We want you to make birdies and pars, but we also want you to be healthy. This chapter includes tips and advice that will not only help you improve your golf game, but also help you maintain a healthy and vigorous lifestyle.

PLAY GOLF, LIVE LONGER

Do you know that playing golf can help you live longer? A study published in the *Scandinavian Journal of Medicine and Science in Sports* conducted by Anders Ahlbom and Bahman Farahmand (2008) at the

Karolinska Institute in Stockholm, Sweden, showed that people who play golf enjoy an increase in life expectancy. It is based on data from 300,000 Swedish golfers. According to the study, the death rate for golfers is 40 percent lower than for nongolfers of the same sex, age, and socioeconomic status. This increased life expectancy could equate to five additional years of life.[1]

The only catch is that the study examined golfers who walked while they played and excluded those who rode in carts. According to Ahlbom, "A round of golf means being outside for four or five hours, walking at a fast pace for about four miles."[2] Other factors, such as a generally healthy lifestyle, may help explain the lower death rate, the scientists said. Ahlbom also says that, "People play golf into old age, and there are also positive social and psychological aspects to the game that can help."[3] It is also likely that playing the game itself has a significant impact on health, so even if you don't walk while you play, playing golf could extend your life.

BREATHING FOR BETTER GOLF

Breathing is our first act in life, as well as our last. For the most part, breathing is an involuntary activity. It is something we do naturally, without thinking. As human beings, it is only a matter of time before we try to take control, as only humans are wont to do, and direct our brain to hold our breath and release it upon direction, at times explosively. Breathing is one of the few bodily functions that, within limits, can be controlled both consciously and subconsciously.

Ever see a dog hold its breath? How about a cat, horse, cow, or wolf? Nope! What about a two-year-old child? Ever see a toddler take a big gulp of air working up to that ear-piercing wail that they know will get your attention? The control pattern starts early in life. Deep breathing, in through the nose and out through open or pursed lips, not only has a positive effect on your game, it has a profound effect on your overall health and well-being. When we breathe, we bring life-giving oxygen into our bodies and force carbon dioxide waste out. Physically speaking, breathing sustains the natural metabolic processes of the body. Psychologically, breathing keeps the mind calm and focused. According to a study in the *British Medical Journal* by Luciano et al., a slow respiratory rate improves cardiovascular and respiratory function, enhances blood oxygenation, elevates exercise tolerance, and increases calmness and well-being.[4]

This all sounds very interesting, but how does any of this affect your golf game? According to Pilates expert and GFM contributor Deanna E. Zenger, breathing has everything to do with golf. When we experience stress on the golf course, whether it is our first shot, a tough lie, or any shot that creates general anxiety, our breathing becomes shallow and erratic.

Golfers hold their breath when they take their swing for many reasons, says Zenger. Driving, chipping, or putting, it doesn't matter. They hold their breath. Holding your breath does not improve your golf swing. In fact, it does the exact opposite. Under pressure, the physiological effect of holding your breath produces a "fight or flight" response in your brain, resulting in a loss of blood flow to the extremities, including the brain. Your body becomes tense, your mind races, and you lose the ability to execute a proper golf swing. Holding your breath also creates tension in your muscles, and when you finally exhale, your body releases a sudden rush of blood throughout your system. The tension in your muscles prevents you from executing the same degree of rotation in your golf swing, says Zenger.

To practice breathing correctly, sit in a chair, relax, and take a nice deep breath in through your nose. Breathe the air all the way in, fully expanding your lungs until you comfortably cannot take in any more. Pause for a moment, and then exhale through parted lips. Your exhalation should be long and slow. Let every last ounce of air and carbon dioxide waste out of your lungs. Gently parting or pursing your lips facilitates a full exhalation. Do this three times, relaxing deeply with each breath.

Deep Breathing to De-stress Your Golf Game

In *Take Control of Your Subconscious Mind* (2000), Anthony T. Gaile agrees with Zenger. He says that psychological stress can be as destructive to the body as physical stress. When an organism is placed under stress, the body goes on alert. The heart rate increases, muscles tense up, blood pressure goes up, and adrenaline begins to flow at a rapid rate. Stress can be whatever the mind perceives it to be, so if you are playing badly and your blood starts to boil because you miss a few short putts or your ball careens off a sprinkler head and into a hazard, you are putting your body under stress.[5]

Periodic breaks in the stress level are needed for the body to be able to reconstruct itself, according to Gaile, otherwise you put yourself at high risk for such problems as tension headaches, stomachaches, fatigue, and even heart attacks, not to mention that your golf game will suffer.[6] For all these reasons, it is important to reduce stress often to let the body rejuvenate itself.

Golf is supposed to be relaxing, but for many people, a missed putt, bad hole, or disappointing round can lead to undue stress and anxiety, causing our breathing to become quick and shallow and depriving our organs of enough oxygen to function properly. Deep breathing releases tension from the body and clears the mind, improving both physical and mental wellness.

The following is another simple, yet effective breathing exercise:

- Stand up straight.
- Exhale completely through your mouth.
- Inhale through your nose, keeping your mouth closed.
- Hold your breath as you count to five.
- Slowly exhale through your mouth for a count of five.

Try this exercise any time you need to relax and release tension.

IS GOLF MAKING YOU FAT?

You may think that you are getting enough exercise while playing golf; however, if you ride in a cart, you are eliminating the benefits of golf as exercise. Add a hot dog, chips, soda, or a couple of beers at the turn, and you may actually be taking in more calories than you are burning.

The best way to get the health benefits that playing golf can provide is to walk while you play. Walking is one of the best activities that people of all ages can do to improve cardiovascular conditioning. A 150-pound person walking at a pace of 4 miles per hour can burn up to 400 calories per hour. Walking 18 or even 9 holes a couple of times a week can help you maintain or even lose weight, as well as boost your endurance, lower your cholesterol, and prevent heart disease. But even if you are required to use a golf cart while you play at your course or you choose not to walk, you can still get exercise during your round by changing a few habits. Try the following calorie-burning and muscle-toning tips the next time you tee it up:

- *Arrive at the golf course with enough time to do a 10-minute warm-up session before you play.* Stretching before you golf loosens your muscles, prepares them for what lies ahead, and can prevent injury.
- *Grab your pitching wedge, 6-iron, and driver and walk to the practice range before your round instead of hopping into the cart and riding*

the few hundred yards. The walk will warm up your muscles and get your heart pumping to improve endurance.

- *Sit up straight and don't slouch while you sit in the cart.* Engage your abdominal muscles, align your head and neck with your spine, and roll your shoulders back to help strengthen the muscles and protect your back. One minute of sitting with the proper posture burns two calories, while sitting with the improper posture burns only one calorie per minute, so with a little extra effort, you can strengthen your abdominal muscles, improve your posture, and burn a few extra calories while you play.
- *Stand up and be ready to hit.* Don't just sit on the cart waiting for your turn. Not only will this speed up play, but standing burns more calories than sitting. Sitting also constricts your muscles and restricts blood flow to them, so they will not respond as well when you swing. As you stand, place a club behind your shoulders to remind you to stand up straight. This is also an excellent way to stretch your back, chest, and shoulders.
- *Stretch between shots.* While you are waiting for the group in front of you to clear the fairway or green, you can do simple stretching exercises to keep your swing loose and supple and increase your flexibility. Stretching also burns more calories than sitting and doing nothing. Take advantage of this down time and work on your flexibility. See chapter 6 for stretches you can do on the golf course.

FITNESS FOR YOUR BRAIN
MENTAL CHALLENGE

To expand your mind, you need to learn new facts and develop new modes of thinking that will make the information that you already know more useful. Puzzles are good for people of all ages because they help sharpen memory and delay the onset of age-related mental disorders. The following is a simple word problem to help you keep your mind as fit as your body.

Harry and Jeff are rehashing their scores after playing a par-five hole. Harry says, "If I had taken one shot less and you had taken one shot more, we would have tied for the hole." Jeff then counters, saying, "Yes, and if I had taken one shot less and you had taken one shot more, you would have taken twice as many shots as me." How many shots did each take?

Solution: Harry took seven shots, and Jeff took five.

IT'S NEVER TOO LATE TO GET YOUR BODY IN GOLF SHAPE

Studies have shown that the senior population actually has a higher potential for strength gains than those in their 20s, 30s, and 40s, primarily due to the lower baseline activity level of the older group. Compared with younger groups performing similar exercises over a one-month period, the aging population can achieve more than double the strength gains of people under age 40. You are never too old to start, and the results can have a dramatic effect on your daily life and your golf game.

If golf is your only form of exercise, you could be doing your golf game and your body a disservice, since the golf swing is a repetitive movement that puts unusual strain on certain parts of the body. The only way to counteract the stress placed on the body and protect yourself from injury is by stretching and strengthening the golf muscles in your neck, back, arms, and legs. Combine the risks of not exercising with the normal effects of decreased strength, flexibility, and rate of healing of body tissues as you age, and you may suddenly be facing injuries that keep you on the recliner rather than the golf cart.

The following are a few facts related to aging:

- *Almost everyone will experience lower back pain at some point in his or her life.* This type of pain is one of the top 10 reasons why people go to see their primary care physicians.
- *Arthritis affects 50 percent of Americans over the age of 65.* It is most common in the hips, spine, and knees. Along with taking medications that your physician may prescribe, eating a healthy diet, maintaining a low body weight, and participating in moderate exercise, including appropriate strengthening and flexibility exercises, can prevent and help manage arthritis.
- *To achieve a normal golf swing, you need good range of motion in your shoulders, spine, and hips.* Limitations in any of these areas will place more strain on other joints and muscles, eventually causing injury. You will also try to overcompensate during your golf swing, which may cause you to hit the ball fat, thin, or just completely off course.

And the following are a few things you can do to ease your aches and pains as you age:

- *Get plenty of exercise.* Increasing your activity level using specific exercises can prevent injury, address current limitations, minimize existing problems, and help fine-tune your golf game. Choose exercises that stretch and strengthen the area where you experience the most limitations. Build up your range of motion, flexibility, and strength by increasing the amount of stretching you do and the number of times you perform each exercise.

- *Do manual therapy.* Some problems require more than just exercise to get your muscles into shape. Oftentimes our joints become tight, and we require specific stretching exercises to target the joint and surrounding areas. Exercises and hands-on techniques performed by a therapist can often lead to the quickest recovery.

- *Get proper hydration and nutrition.* Both are important regardless of age. Without the proper foundation of a well-balanced diet and fluid intake, your body cannot function at its best, no matter what your fitness level. Try eating a small, healthy snack (for example, yogurt or a small apple with peanut butter) about an hour or two before working out to ensure that you have enough energy to get you through your workout. Also make sure that you drink plenty of water while on the course or driving range.

Following the guidelines presented in this book can help you maintain and even improve your golf swing as you get older. Prevention is always the best way to stay healthy and active as you age.

....

PLAYING GOLF CAN LOWER YOUR RISK OF STROKE

Men and women with moderate levels of cardiovascular fitness may be able to significantly reduce their risk of a stroke, according to a new study presented at the International Stroke Conference in 2008. It is well-documented that regular exercise and related fitness enhances cardiovascular health. Golf, a low-impact sport, may be a great way to help people not only improve overall health, but also reduce their risk of suffering a stroke.

According to the study, those who participate in any kind of physical activity that meets the current guidelines and recommendations for adults, for example, brisk walking for 30 minutes 3 times per week, can significantly reduce their stroke risk. Golf can be good for your health and safe for your heart, but these health benefits don't come from swinging a club, they come from walking. Since trekking across the average course for a round of golf can equate to as much as 4 miles of walking, if you walk 18 holes 3 to 5 times a week, you can get the optimal amount of endurance exercise for your heart. If you pull your clubs or carry them, you'll burn even more calories per round and benefit even more.

GET ORGANIZED FOR BETTER SCORES

Do you know that your chaotic routine and cluttered golf bag might be holding you back from playing your best golf? Nothing is more frustrating and stressful than standing on the first tee and having people waiting for you to tee off while you rifle through your golf bag looking for a glove, ball, or tee. Everyone can benefit from a more organized golf bag, which can help you play faster and eliminate stress.

The following are a few suggestions to help you organize your golf bag.

- *Clean out your golf bag every few weeks.* Throw out old golf balls, worn out gloves, broken tees, half-eaten protein bars, empty golf ball boxes, and old sunscreen bottles and lip balms.
- *Separate and organize your golf accessories.* Keep your golf balls, gloves, tees, and ball markers in separate pockets. Use the big pockets in your bag for your golf balls and the smaller ones for tees and ball markers. Avoid dumping everything in one pocket.
- *Keep your tees and ball markers in clear plastic baggies.* This allows you to easily see what you are looking for and avoid dumping the entire contents of your bag on the ground just to find your favorite ball marker or the correct size tee.
- *Throw away those old, dirty golf towels hanging on your golf bag.* Not only are they unsightly, they are hotbeds for bacteria and germs. Replace and wash your towel often. Do not let it become the next *CSI: Miami* episode.
- *Purchase a new golf bag with easy-to-access pockets and club organizers.* Newer golf bags have more pockets and compartments, so you can organize your golf accessories and better protect your equipment.

....

■ Ladies Tee
OSTEOPOROSIS AND GOLF

Due to a large aging population, osteoporosis is reaching epidemic proportions and is responsible for more than 1.5 million fractures annually. Based on figures from hospitals and nursing homes, the national direct expenditure for osteoporosis and osteoporosis-related fractures totals $14 billion each year.[7] According to the World Health Organization, osteoporosis is second only to cardiovascular disease as a leading health care problem. In Europe and the United States combined, the lifetime risk of hip fracture in women is greater than the sum of lifetime risks of breast, endometrial, and ovarian cancer. Globally, one out of every two women and one out of every five men is affected by the condition.[8]

Implementing an exercise program can help prevent or treat osteoporosis by increasing muscle strength, maintaining bone density, and improving balance to help avoid falls. According to the Mayo Foundation for Medical Education and Research, golf can provide beneficial exercise for most people with osteoporosis.[9] With proper mechanics, golf can help place appropriate stress on bones to help them maintain density and strength.

EXERCISING WITH A COLD OR THE FLU

Deciding whether to work out when you don't feel well can be a difficult decision. You want to stay in shape, but you also don't want to make yourself sicker. The following are a few guidelines from the Aerobic and Fitness Association of America to help you decide whether to work out:

- *Check with your physician to see if it is safe for you to exercise while you are sick*. It is not a good idea to further endanger your health if you are ill.
- *Consider others*. If you are contagious, you should probably skip going to the gym, where you could contaminate other people.
- *Consider the risks of exercising while you are sick*. One major risk is heat stroke and heat exhaustion. When you are sick or feverish, the body cannot deal with overheating as well as usual; therefore, you run an increased risk of heat stroke, which can be fatal. Another major risk is the potential for developing a viral infection. According to Dr. David Schechter, a sports medicine specialist, viral infections can lead to heart failure and even death. Although this condition is rare, it is best to avoid overexerting yourself. Exercising when you are sick may make your condition worse. If you have bronchitis, for example, according to Dr. Schechter, the stress of exercise and temporary dip in the immune system that has been documented to occur with strenuous exercise could lead to a worsening of the bronchitis or the development of pneumonia, a serious lung infection.[10]
- *Use common sense when you are sick and considering working out*. Avoid exercise when you experiencing a fever, muscle aches, shakes, chills, or vomiting. These symptoms are often present when a viral or bacterial infection is at its peak.

Although a quick workout while you are sick may be a temporary pick-me-up, avoiding exercising while you are sick may be your best bet for a speedy recovery.

SLEEP BETTER TO IMPROVE YOUR GAME

Your best source of energy is sleep. Inadequate sleep is associated with heart disease, diabetes, and obesity. Studies show that eight hours of sleep a night is ideal for optimal health. Sleeping better will not only give you more energy on the golf course, it will keep you alert and enable you to concentrate for the four to five hours that it takes to play. The following are a few tips to help you sleep better:

- *Replace old bedding.* Throw out mattresses that are more than 10 years old. Mattresses lose firmness after years of wear. Throw out pillows that are more than three years old. Pillows collect bacteria and dust mites that can make people sick. Wash your sheets often, and toss your pillows into the dryer each month to kill dust mites.
- *Turn off the television and computer.* Watching television or working on the computer before you go to bed can stimulate your brain and make it hard for you to relax and unwind.
- *Keep the noise level down in your bedroom.* Use a fan or white noise machine to block outside noise. Dim the lights half an hour before going to bed to signal your brain that it is time to rest.
- *Exercise regularly.* Performing just 20 to 30 minutes of exercise per day can help improve sleep. Just be sure to exercise in the morning or early afternoon. Avoid exercising late in the day, as it will stimulate your body and make it harder for you to fall asleep.

LAUGH YOUR WAY TO A BETTER GAME

Golf is a sport that requires a lot of focus, concentration, and mental stamina. Anyone who has cracked up at a joke or watched a funny movie knows that laughing makes you feel better, but do you know that research shows that laughter can strengthen your immune system, help you tolerate pain better, and even make you smarter? According to Michael Lovorn, a humor researcher and education teacher at California State University, Long Beach, "Laughing contributes to a good mind and body balance." Having a good belly laugh every once in a while can help boost your memory and relieve stress.

THINGS TO CONSIDER WHEN HIRING A GOLF FITNESS TRAINER

If you are in the market for a personal trainer to help you improve your golf fitness, there are a few things to take into consideration, says Peter Kadzielawski, co-owner of Equilibrium Personal Training. "Your new trainer should be certified, but please understand that a certification is not everything. Just because you have a driver's license does not make you a great driver," says Kadzielawski.

According to Kadzielawski, you do have to go through a tough program and pass a test to get certified, but the certification is basically a license for someone to legally call himself or herself a personal trainer. Consider hiring a personal trainer who is certified in golf fitness. Your trainer does not have to be a golf guru or expert, but he or she should understand the basic fundamentals of the swing and the importance of balance, coordination, and flexibility in golf.

Kadzielawski has a few suggestions for hiring your next personal trainer. First and foremost, your trainer should be fit and have several years of experience training people. If someone can keep himself or herself in great shape, it increases the chances that he or she will be able to help you. A personal level of fitness demonstrates that they themselves have a personal understanding of what it takes to stay fit.

You should also look for a trainer with many years of experience and references to prove it. Someone who has been achieving great results with their clients won't have a problem providing that information. Don't hesitate to contact a previous client to see what their experience with that particular trainer was like. Your trainer should be able to show you how working on core flexibility and specific shoulder strengthening exercises and stretches improved their previous client's golf game.

Second, Kadzielawski says that a great fitness professional will offer a free consultation or orientation session to take the time to get to know you. The first time you meet your potential trainer, he or she should sit down with you and find out as much as they can about you. It is a promising sign when the trainer asks questions about you, your lifestyle, and your goals, rather than talking about how much they know about general fitness and trying to impress or overwhelm you with random information. For example, many golfers suffer from lower back pain, and your new instructor should find out if you are one of them. If you do suffer from this type of discomfort, your trainer should share some ways to strengthen your lower back and stretching exercises that can help you.

He or she should also stress the importance of strengthening your abdominal muscles and explain how this can help take the pressure off of your lower back and increase the range of motion in your golf swing. At this time, your trainer should establish a plan to help you improve your fitness and explain in simple terms how he or she will help you meet your goals through specific exercises that will not only challenge your balance, but also work on your coordination and increase your strength.

Finally, the orientation session is your last chance to figure out if he or she is the right trainer for you, says Kadzielawski. If 15 minutes into your orientation session you are out of breath and really hating it, this trainer may not be for you. The trainer may simply lack experience. A great personal trainer with the proper education and experience will not "beat you up" during your first workout, even if you are a very fit person.

If you are a golf-specific client, your first session should be educational and include a golf-specific fitness screen and low- to medium-intensity exercises. Your instructor should ensure that you understand the basics and be clear about why he or she is choosing this type of routine for your first workout. At the end of the orientation session, if you feel a little tired, but also like you have been educated, inspired, and motivated, and you even had a little fun, congratulations, you have found the person who can lead you to an amazing life change and improve your golf game in the process.

TRY A GOLF-SPECIFIC MASSAGE TO RELIEVE PAIN

As a massage therapist, a GFM contributor, and an avid golfer, Lisa Ferguson is acutely aware of the physical tolls of the game, because most of her clients are golfers. "To play a good game of golf, you must be fit to play well. What does being fit really mean? It means being healthy. Being fit means that your muscle tissues need to be healthy, flexible and mobile. Healthy muscle tissues have the ability to create efficient spontaneous movements and prevent injuries. That's why spas offering golf-specific massages are on the rise. It is important to knead out those aches and pains that are so specific to golfers," says Ferguson.

How does soreness affect a golfer's swing? Think about having a sore back. It is uncomfortable to walk, stand, sit, and sometimes even touch the affected area. When muscle tissues are sore, they are weak and under stress and need specific massage-related therapies. A golfer's swing is unnatural to the body because of the fact that you must be in a slightly bending position while trying to hit the ball. The swing involves a stance that requires you to shift your weight from the left to the right to the left again, which demands flexibility in the hips, while at the same time winding your upper back in a coiling movement while your hips stay balanced beneath you. If your back is sore, your muscles cannot perform efficiently, and you risk further injury, like a lumbar sprain or strain.

How Many Golfers Are Suffering?

More than 50 percent of golfers suffer from neck weakness, lower back problems, shoulder or rotator cuff stiffness, elbow dysfunction, lower leg imbalances, and/or wrist injuries. If a golfer continues playing with stiffness and soreness in the back, further injury to surrounding muscle groups is a risk. This can result in chronic pain cycles, which will interfere with enjoyment of the game. That is where golf massage comes into play.

Massage Therapy for Golfers

Massage can help people from all walks of life, but for the athlete or weekend golfer, it can relax tension and relieve painful, sore, and stiff muscles. If you are experiencing soreness, stiffness, or pain, regular therapeutic massage can help you get relief and improve your game. Massage allows for the reprogramming of the nervous system and opens channels for new habits to form. If you are receiving training lessons, massage can keep muscles less stressed and better able to adopt new strategies to help better your swing.

Massage also promotes health, vitality, and well-being. It allows for the release of muscular tension and stress, eliminates metabolic waste products, and restores muscle elasticity, length, and range of motion. Massage has positive physiological effects on the nervous system and organs as well. It releases powerful endorphins that give you a great feeling after a rub down.

HOW GOLF-SPECIFIC MASSAGE CAN REDUCE THE RISK OF INJURY

Golfers are less likely to incur injuries if their muscles are flexible and mobile. Massage can be especially beneficial if you are returning to the game after a long hiatus and are looking to get your muscles moving again.

Golf massage is also specifically designed to work all of the muscle groups involved in the swing. Healthy muscles help maintain communication between themselves and the nervous system. This enables efficient movement of the muscles controlling the extremities, as well as those controlling your center of gravity, or your core. This movement is key in maintaining the dynamic balance required for a proper golf swing. Healthy muscles also help preserve bone structure to ensure good posture.

TYPES OF MASSAGE THERAPY

There are relaxation massages and therapeutic massages. A relaxation massage involves touch with light to moderate pressure. It involves continuous strokes and a rhythmic gliding touch that creates a total-body experience. Examples include Swedish and Esalen massages, which use effleurage, pettrissage, and kneading.

Therapeutic massages are best for golfers, because they address the specific muscles that tend to tighten from play or overuse. The following are four different therapeutic massages and what they accomplish to help relieve stress and restore your aching muscles.

1. *Deep-tissue massage therapy combines deep pressure with kneading strokes to help relieve tight muscles and connective tissues.* This type of massage focuses on muscle tension to help release the toxins that cause muscles stiffness.

2. *Myofascial trigger point therapy releases the triggers that limit the range of motion of the muscle.* These triggers can also cause pain, myofascial dysfunction, soreness, and stiffness.

3. *Sports massage therapy pairs rigorous massaging strokes with passive assisted stretching to relax tightened muscles.* When performed on a regular basis, this type of massage can help prevent injury by improving muscle condition.

4. *Neuromuscular therapy restores elasticity in the muscle fibers by stripping and breaking up adhesions caused by injuries or muscle strains.* This type of therapy helps stabilize low levels of neurological activity to maintain normal function and overall health.

Ferguson highly recommends these types of massage because the results are enormously effective for the golfer. Regaining flexibility, mobility, and stability in the hips, shoulders, legs, and arms are a must in improving your body's ability to perform a great golf swing. Ferguson uses a combination of these therapies, depending on the client's issues and goals.

"My treatment goals must be in line with what the client wants from their sessions—decreased pain, more range of motion, or stability and balance. My success partially depends upon the client too, and whether they are consistent with their treatments and stretching/strengthening programs. Overall, most of my clients become pain free, and after the first few sessions, golfers report benefits like their drive was much better, their back didn't hurt to swing the club, or they noticed improvement in their ball striking ability. Receiving specific attention to the muscle groups used in a swing is important because a golfer can gain more power, more distance, and better endurance," says Ferguson.

WHAT YOU NEED TO KNOW ABOUT MINIMALLY INVASIVE SPINE SURGERY

According to internationally renowned neurosurgeon and GFM contributor Dr. Robert Masson, minimally invasive spine surgery techniques have gained much attention in the last several years, yet more often than not, many patients do not really understand the good, the bad, and the ugly when it comes to making their own treatment decisions. The bottom line is that the most important question regarding a proposed procedure and its benefit is, "does the surgery hit the target?" says Masson. That is when minimally invasive technology becomes important. And as an educated patient, you need to know a little bit about the tools, the philosophy, and the marketing.

Many tools are useful in minimally invasive spine surgery. Everyone knows about lasers, endoscopes, microscopes, and so on and so forth. But it is also important to understand that each tool has a benefit when used properly, and the benefits vary depending on the skill set of the surgeon using them. In other words, when you read about the miraculous benefits of laser surgery, you must understand that a surgeon still needs to get the laser to the intended target, and it is this access that defines minimally invasive approaches.

When a surgeon discusses a proposed minimally invasive procedure, it is not the tool used in dealing with a herniated disc, but the amount of retraction, the volume of soft tissue damage, the accuracy of the approach, and the efficiency of movement that defines the procedure as minimally invasive. Do not be dazzled by the technology. Rather, focus on the strategy being discussed when you choose a minimally invasive procedure, says Masson.

Minimally invasive surgery is a philosophy, not an approach. A well-rounded and competent spine surgeon uses a variety of approaches and has numerous tools. He or she can approach the spine from the front, the back, or the side, but it is choosing the best approach with the least resulting trauma that defines a procedure as minimally invasive. The philosophy of minimally invasive spine surgery provides that all approaches be done with minimal trauma and maximal benefit. This type of surgery goes wrong when it is minimal strategy surgery, or when the goals are sacrificed to achieve the outcome. It is crucial that the goals of the surgery be understood and that there is a statistically significant chance of achieving the desired outcome. A thoughtful minimally invasive approach involves the highest sophistication in preoperative diagnosis and planning and requires that significant effort is made by the surgical team to understand the problem; the symptoms, the patient's needs, expectations, and goals; and ultimately the liabilities as they relate to each individual patient.

There are many multibillion dollar medical device companies manufacturing and marketing the tools and devices for these procedures. These include artificial discs, retractor systems, endoscopes, and lasers. Do not be afraid to ask how each surgeon uses these devices, how many surgeries they have done, whether they are limited to one approach, and how they plan to use their tools to help you get results, continues Masson.

It is important that you as the patient make your own choices based on your relationship with the surgeon, and your trust in his or her abilities and reputation. If it does not feel like a good fit, find a surgeon who gives you that feeling. You will be the one who has to live with the effects of the chosen surgery for the rest of your life.

SUMMARY

Being fit can reduce the risks of obesity, osteoporosis, diabetes, heart disease, high blood pressure, and stroke, but it can also help us boost our immune system to prevent illness and injury and relieve stress. For those of us who love to play golf, being fit is crucial in performing at our best on the golf course and finding more enjoyment in the game. Many professional golfers have been doing golf-specific training and getting phenomenal results for years, and recreational golfers are finally jumping on the bandwagon to enhance their games and longevity. We at GFM believe that golf-specific fitness is the key to improved performance.

Although Tiger Woods didn't invent golf fitness (it is a well-known fact that Gary Player practiced fitness early in his career and that the PGA Tour and LPGA Tour have had fitness trailers and trainers at Tour events since the mid-1980s), he has helped spread the word since bursting onto the golf scene in 1996 and kicking it up a notch with his golf-specific training. Woods has clearly demonstrated how being fit for golf can elevate one's game.

Following Tiger's lead, golf professionals now work out like elite athletes. Golf fitness has gained popularity and is now a staple on all the professional golf tours. In addition, studies have been done on the biomechanics of golf and the effects of the golf swing on the body. Many industry professionals have been gathering data from touring pros and have used that data to more clearly define the positive impact of fitness on golf. The evidence is clear: Golf Fitness is beneficial. Our goal at GFM is and has been to expose golfers of all levels to golf fitness and related topics, like the mental side of the game, injury prevention, nutrition, and longevity.

Anyone who plays golf, whether professionally, competitively in club leagues, or casually, understands the physical demands of the game. The load placed on the body while in full swing is tremendous, and even practicing long and short games can wreak havoc on a player's back. So how can we alleviate pain or mitigate the impact on the body? We can do it through golf-specific fitness.

Golf fitness is not just exercise. Being fit for golf includes choosing the right foods, thinking the right thoughts, and learning to relax and enjoy the game. We hope that this book has given you ideas about how to improve your swing and score, but also about how to be healthier. Golf-specific fitness can help golfers of all levels with their game, not only reducing their handicap and improving their golf playing abilities, but also extending their playing career and preventing injury.

So how does being fit for golf translate to improving your game? The full swing is an unnatural movement carried out at a very high rate of speed, and the stress that the body goes through is unique to the swing. Understanding how those stresses affect the musculoskeletal system is important in defining a golf fitness program. Just as every player is unique, so too should be a golf fitness program.

As we have stated in previous chapters, before you embark on a golf-specific fitness program, begin with a physical assessment. The assessment will help determine your areas of weakness, specifically areas of concern regarding balance, mobility, stability, and flexibility. A player should be strong but also have enough flexibility and stability to repeatedly perform the rigors of a golf swing without pain or injury. An assessment can help determine your unique problem areas.

Once your areas of weakness have been determined, a program can be designed to address those concerns. We have provided numerous examples of exercises that can correct physical swing limitations. When a golfer has physical limitations, he or she is forced to make compensations in the golf swing, which, besides causing errant shots, can lead to acute and chronic injury. A high-handicap player is at greater risk of injury. But with a proper assessment and an exercise program prescribed to help strengthen, stretch, and address the player's weaknesses, a golfer can improve.

Our approach is a different way to learn the game of golf. We believe that fundamentals and swing mechanics are interconnected and important to the game, but we also know that improving your body and mind will enable you to play better golf. To accelerate your improvement process, consider hiring a golf fitness professional or golf teacher certified in golf fitness to help guide you through a program. This is the best way to get your game on track. A golf coach/instructor can identify your swing faults and relay the information to the trainer, and the trainer can screen you for physical limitations.

Being fit for golf is a lifestyle that encompasses golf-specific exercise, nutrition, and the mental aspects of the game. Committing to making such small changes in your daily routine as stretching for a few minutes, adding a few strength and balance exercises to your fitness routine, choosing fruit over a candy bar, and managing your thoughts differently on the course can tremendously enhance your game. A bonus is being a healthier individual.

NOTES

CHAPTER 3
ASSESSING YOUR GOLF ABILITY

1. The basic golf-specific screen is designed for any golfer who is trying to determine his or her level of golf fitness or planning to start a golf-specific training program. If you are currently injured or have any medical problems, consult your physician before attempting this screen and/or any exercise program. This screen is in no way meant to diagnose medical conditions but rather to assess physical limitations and establish baseline measurements to establish a functional golf conditioning program for people who have received medical clearance from their physicians. Consult either a golf fitness professional or teaching professional certified in golf fitness for a complete evaluation.

2. Plyometric exercises involve an increased risk of injury due to the large forces generated during training and performance and should only be performed by well-conditioned individuals who are under the supervision of a trained professional.

CHAPTER 8
PILATES AND YOGA FOR GOLF

1. Lieber, Jill, "Male Athletes Get No Pain, Big Gains from Pilates." [Online article, 2009, n.p.] Accessed September 10, 2010, from www.usatoday.com/sports/2003-08-17-pilates_x.htm.

CHAPTER 9
NUTRITION FOR GOLF

1. Henneman, Alice, "Nuts for Nutrition" [Online article, 2009.] Accessed September 10, 2010, from http://lancaster.unl.edu/food/ftmar04.htm.

CHAPTER 10
THE MENTAL GAME

1. Nicklaus, Jack, with Ken Bowen, *Golf My Way* (New York: Simon & Schuster, 1974).

CHAPTER 11
THE HEALTHY GOLFER

1. Farahmand, Bahman, and Anders Ahlbom, "Golf, a Game of Life and Death: Reduced Mortality in Swedish Golf Players." *Scandinavian Journal of Medicine and Science in Sports.* [Online article, 28 May 2008.] DOI: 10.1111/j.1600-0838.2008.00814.x.

2. Farahmand and Ahlbom, "Golf, a Game of Life and Death," n.p.

3. Farahmand and Ahlbom, "Golf, a Game of Life and Death," n.p.

4. Bernardi, Luciano, Peter Sleight, Gabriele Bandinelli, Simone Cencetti, Lamberto Fattorini, Johanna Wdowczyc-Szulc, and Alfonso Lagi, "Beyond Science: The Effect of Rosary Prayer and Yoga Mantras on Autonomic Cardiovascular Rhythms." *British Medical Journal, 323* (December 2001): 22–29.

5. Gaile, Anthony T., *Take Control of Your Subconscious Mind* (Chicago: Cornerstone Press, 2000).

6. Gaile, *Take Control of Your Subconscious Mind.*

7. eMedTV, "Osteoporosis Research." [Online article, 2009.] Accessed September 10, 2010, from http://osteoporosis.emedtv.com/osteoporosis/osteoporosis-research.html.

8. World Health Organization, "Attacking Pain via Acupuncture." *Acupuncture and Pain Management Journal*, 26 (May 2008): A43.

9. Mayo Foundation for Medical Education and Research, "Exercise: Seven Benefits of Regular Physical Activity." [Online article, 2009.] Accessed September 10, 2010, from www.mayoclinic.com/health/exercise/HQ01676.

10. Aerobics and Fitness Association of America, "Fitness Gets Personal." [Online article, 2009.] Accessed September 10, 2010, from http://www.afaa.com/.

INDEX

ABOUT THE CONTRIBUTORS

Karen Palacios-Jansen is managing editor of GFM. She was voted the 2008 LPGA National Teacher of the Year and is a CHEK certified golf performance specialist and a certified personal trainer. Palacios-Jansen is also a frequently requested public speaker and lecturer at local and national golf shows and conferences and a GFM Advisory Team member.

GOLF FITNESS MAGAZINE ADVISORY TEAM

Erin Booker, MPT, MTC, CSCS, is a GFM Advisory Team member and clinic director for Physiotherapy Associates in Ocoee, Florida.

Brad Brewer is a PGA class-A professional and owner of The Brad Brewer Golf Academy. He was chosen as the North Florida PGA Teacher of the Year and inducted as a Top 100 Teacher in America by *Golf Magazine*. Brewer is also a frequent contributor to The Golf Channel.

Susan Choi graduated from Wellesley College, where she played varsity golf. Choi was chosen from thousands of professional and amateur golfers worldwide to compete on The Golf Channel's reality show *The Big Break Ka'anapali* at Maui's Ka'anapali Resort.

Laura Cippola is founder of Golf Fitness International, where she works with professional, collegiate, and amateur golfers. She is also a contributing writer for GFM and director of education/player development for the Orlando Executive Women's Golf Association.

Sean Cochran is one of the most recognized golf fitness trainers in the world. He travels the PGA Tour working with PGA professionals, most notably two-time Masters and PGA champion Phil Mickelson.

Brett Cook, MS, CSCS, USAW, is professor of exercise science at Palm Beach Atlantic University. She is also a golf performance specialist at PGA National Resort.

Lisa Ferguson is a licensed massage therapist who currently owns and operates Massage Fitness Co. in San Francisco, California.

Roger Fredericks has developed a golf swing and flexibility program that is practiced by some of the greatest names in the sport, including Arnold Palmer and Gary Player. His program is geared toward recreational players hoping to increase their competitiveness and has helped thousands of players improve their game.

Randy Friedman is a motivational speaker, a professional golfer, and the author of *Golf Mind Power*.

Kai Fusser was born in Germany and is director of fitness for the prestigious ANNIKA Academy™ in Orlando, Florida.

Tara Gidus, MS, RD, CSSD, is a board-certified specialist in sports dietetics, nutrition consultant, and member of the GFM Advisory Team.

Steve Gomen is publisher and president of GFM.

Dave Herman is founder of Athleticity Professional. He is also a sports performance coach and an elite tennis player. Herman earned his bachelor's degree in exercise science from the University of South Carolina and is dedicated to helping golfers to improve both their physical and mental games. His clients include professional golfers Ernie Els, Trevor Immelman, Suzann Pettersen, and Skip Kendall.

Kristi Karst-Gomen is senior editor of GFM. She is a former editor of *Lifestyle Publications* and is currently president of Palm Tree Media, as well as the NeuroSpine Institute Foundation, a not-for-profit organization. Karst-Gomen holds a master's degree in journalism.

Robert Masson, MD, is a GFM Advisory Team member. Dr. Masson's practice is devoted to the treatment of spinal disorders and surgery. He is also an international consultant for minimally invasive neurosurgery.

Bill McInerney Jr. has been a professional golf performance coach since 1994. He is certified by the Titleist Performance Institute and is founder of mygolfinggoals.com.

Rob Mottram is a GFM contributor, Titleist Performance Institute advisor, and owner/operator of the Golf Health and Performance Center at Mission Hills Country Club in Rancho Mirage, California.

Katherine Roberts is founder and president of Yoga for Golfers International. She is an expert on yoga and golf and a GFM Advisory Team member.

Donald Wallace holds a doctorate in chiropractics from New York Chiropractic College. He also has an MBA from Long Island University as a mechanical engineer and is certified in spinal rehabilitation from Villanova University. Wallace is the inventor of the GreenStick.

Bob Winters, MD, is considered one of the sport's best sports psychologists and metal conditioning coaches. Dr. Winters has worked with some of the PGA's most successful professionals, as well as more than a dozen NCAA golf teams.

TOUR PROFESSIONAL ADVISORY TEAM

Stuart Appleby is a PGA Tour player and winner of 15 professional events, including 9 wins on the PGA Tour.

Nick Faldo is a PGA Tour player and winner of 40 professional events, including 6 major championships.

Trevor Immelman is a PGA Tour player and winner of 10 professional events, including the 2008 Masters.

Phil Mickelson is a PGA Tour player and winner of 46 professional events, including 4 major championships.

Suzann Pettersen, after her rookie year in 2003, has gone on to win 5 tournaments and earn almost $3 million in winnings. She has twice represented the Jr. Ryder Cup team for Europe.

Justin Rose is a PGA Tour player and winner of seven professional events.